Harmony: Professional Renewal for Nurses

Catherine D. Buckley and Diane Walker
The Einstein Consulting Group,
a subsidiary of Albert Einstein Healthcare Foundation

Judy Stofman, Editor

Bill,

WE COULD NOT HAVE DONE THIS WITHOUT YOUR SUPPORT AND COMMITMENT. HOPE YOU LIKE IT!! PLEASE KEEP THE VISION & SPARK ALIVE. TO A FUTURE TOAST!

Diane and
Katie

AHA®
American Hospital Publishing, Inc.,
a wholly owned subsidiary of the
American Hospital Association

The views expressed in this book are those of the authors.

Library of Congress Cataloging-in-Publication Data

Buckley, Catherine D.
    Harmony: professional renewal for nurses.

        1. Nurses—Job satisfaction. I. Walker, Diane.
II. Stofman, Judy. III. Title. [DNLM: 1. Adaptation,
Psychological. 2. Nursing. 3. Stress, Psychological—
prevention & control. WY 87 B924c]
RT82.B79   1989   610.73'069   88-35017
ISBN 1-55648-029-6

Catalog no. 154150

Text set in Bookman Light
4M—3/89—0230

Audrey Kaufman, Project Editor
Linda Conheady, Manuscript Editor
Marcia Bottoms, Managing Editor
Peggy DuMais, Production Coordinator
Marcia Vecchione, Designer
Joseph S. Kulka, Illustrator
Brian Schenk, Books Division Director

Contents

About the Authors

Catherine D. Buckley, M.S., is director of human resources development services for The Einstein Consulting Group in Philadelphia. She is the recipient of two achievement awards from the Hospital Association of Pennsylvania for exemplary health care staff training. She is the codeveloper of HARMONY, a comprehensive renewal program for nurses, and HOSPITALity, an organizationwide strategy for health care service excellence, and her specialties include management development, team building, and organizational change strategy. She has a master's degree in humanistic education from Marywood College and more than 10 years of experience working with hospitals and other health care organizations nationwide. Before joining The Einstein Consulting Group, she was a director of medical social work.

Diane Walker, M.S.N., is director of nurse development services for The Einstein Consulting Group. Codirector of HARMONY, Ms. Walker has 18 years of experience in the health care field, including 15 years in administrative positions. Formerly director of nursing services for Albert Einstein Medical Center, Northern Division, a 600-bed acute care hospital in Philadelphia, she has also served on the faculty of Ohio State University College of Nursing. She has a bachelor's degree in nursing from Duke University and a master's degree in psychiatric nursing from Rutgers University. Ms. Walker is currently completing a master's degree in business administration from LaSalle University. She has a private practice in psychotherapy and has served as a board member for women's organizations. She is recognized as a charismatic trainer and is noted for her practical knowledge and hands-on experience in the health care field.

List of Figures

Acknowledgments

As we begin to think of all the people to whom we would like to express our heartfelt appreciation for their support, suggestions, and hard work in making this book possible, our list only continues to grow.

First, we would like to thank the nurses of Albert Einstein Medical Center, Northern Division, in Philadelphia, and the hundreds of staff nurses around the country who shared with us their real feelings about what it's like to be a nurse in today's health care environment and what they need most to fulfill their professional role. The one-to-one interviews with nurses around the country, the many focus groups, and our seminars provided the raw material and set the foundation for this book. For this, we thank all those wonderful nurses who participated, cooperated, and gave to us much more than we gave to them.

We would like to thank Wendy Leebov, president of The Einstein Consulting Group, our teacher, friend, and visionary leader, for her empowerment, love, and unwavering encouragement and support. It is her efforts that brought this manuscript to the attention of American Hospital Publishing, Inc.

Bill Warfel, associate general director of Albert Einstein Medical Center, provided endless support and counsel during the exciting evolution of the HARMONY program, and we thank him especially for his willingness to invest in the individual well-being of his staff nurses. He is a true friend.

We would also like to thank the following people:

Judy Stofman, our editor, whose excellent ideas and sparkling writing ability assisted us throughout the development of this book.

We'll never forget the boost we received when Judy came on board and expressed her strong personal belief in our concepts and material and told us we had the makings of a great book. She gave us the confidence to pursue publication.

Silvia Blois, our editorial assistant, for being superb to work with. Her professional standards of excellence and mastery of word processing kept our manuscript alive and looking good, edit after edit.

Ester Love, for her support and for her belief in and long-term commitment to making HARMONY a priority in nursing staff development.

Nida Quirong, Geri Weideman, Gary Bilski, Julie Hensler-Cullen, Ann Marie Mayer, and Sandy Pajka, for being the greatest of nurse managers. They kept the ship floating while we pioneered the way for HARMONY.

Trish Heck and Pat Osborne, who kept the embers burning on the meaningful issue of empathy for patients.

The entire, talented staff of the The Einstein Consulting Group, who rode the roller coaster with us. They shared our daily trials, joys, and celebrations.

Gail Scott, whose astute ability to laser in on the real issues through the world of theater greatly influenced and shaped the life of HARMONY, the program.

Berry, Beth, and "Mr." Nicholas, our loved ones, for renewing our spirits daily, and for putting up with us when we were less than delightful.

To our parents, Dorothy and Maurice Buckley (deceased) and Betty and David Walker (both deceased) for their beautiful gifts of home, family, and faith. And a special acknowledgment for Katie's mother, a nurse whose humanism for patients served as a fountain of inspiration.

To Katie's brothers and sisters, Peter, Ellen, Tim, Ann, and Jerry, for standing behind her the whole way, and for their tremendous capacity for caring.

And to all of the patients we've cared for and cared about, you've been the greatest teachers and sources of fulfillment.

Introduction

Nursing has always been hard work. But in today's health care environment, it is harder than ever. There are cutbacks in funding, difficult government regulations, and the worst nursing shortage in history. All these add up to nurses being challenged to work more effectively than ever and to achieve job satisfaction in an atmosphere of tremendous pressure and shrinking support. Cost-saving measures may be crucial to an organization's survival, but to the nursing staff they mean stress, frustration, and attrition.

With job stress high and morale at an all-time low, inter-departmental tensions have grown to epidemic proportions. With fewer nurses on staff and with the budgetary scalpel cutting deep, nurses are expected to do more with less—work more shifts, attend more and sicker patients, and perform a broader range of duties. And they're expected to do all this with greater sensitivity, patience, and empathy. It is ironic that the emphasis on patient satisfaction in health care comes at a time when the pressures are making high-quality care next to impossible—when "safe care" has become the motto of many nurses. One inevitable result of all of these pressures and demands is the increased danger of professional burnout.

The prospect sounds really dismal, doesn't it? Well, it's far from hopeless. Even in these difficult and frustrating times, you can take time out and look more closely at the career you've chosen and realize your desire for greater satisfaction, fulfillment, and joy in your professional life. We'd like to help you do just that.

What Is the Professional Renewal Approach?

The Professional Renewal concept is grounded in three fundamental principles:

- **Principle 1: You are responsible for your own job satisfaction.** You can satisfy yourself by making active choices among the many alternatives available to you. This involves taking charge of yourself and committing yourself to taking actions that make you happy. In this book, we stress *choice* on almost every page. Many choices are available to you at any given moment, even during trying circumstances. Our approach focuses inward on the internal world you control, rather than outward on the external world that you cannot control. Professional Renewal is about choosing—choosing enabling thoughts, feelings, and actions over self-defeating thoughts, feelings, and actions; choosing health over tension and illness; choosing happiness over unhappiness.
- **Principle 2: You need to see your work and your life as expressions of energy.** All that we think, feel, and do expresses our own inner life energy. How are you spending it? Wasting it? Stifling it? How can you take in more life-giving energy, magnify it, and multiply it? Professional Renewal is designed to help unleash that energy to live by, that energy to work by.
- **Principle 3: You have powerful intuition and a sense of what's good for you at any given moment. You have the power to make yourself happy.** This book is designed to help you listen to and trust your own inner wisdom. For some of us, this inner wisdom is a language once understood, but now out of reach. We've all experienced those moments when we fumed and frustrated ourselves instead of speaking up, when we blew up or broke down instead of breaking through, when we got stuck in "ain't it awfuls" and chronic complaining that sapped our energy reserves for the day.

Instead of ignoring, resisting, or submerging this inner guidance, Professional Renewal helps to reestablish that communication between you and your instincts about what's good for you. Nurses struggle with tough questions:

- How can I gain a greater sense of control over the incredible demands on me?
- How can I feel a greater sense of accomplishment and success?
- How can I find greater satisfaction and rewards?

- How do I know if I'm cut out to be a nurse? Is all the stress and strain worth it?

This approach helps you to look inside for the answers. The solutions are there.

The Story of Harmony

In our work at The Albert Einstein Consulting Group, helping hospitals nationwide excel in service dimensions, we learned of the mounting frustration and job dissatisfaction on the part of many, many nurses. Overwhelmed, angry, highly stressed, anxious, disenchanted, disillusioned, depressed—these were words used repeatedly to describe the nurse's plight. Short of changing the entire health care system, we decided to dedicate ourselves to helping nurses achieve satisfaction and fulfillment in their important work.

Around the same time, the nursing service department at the Albert Einstein Medical Center in Philadelphia established a departmental objective of strengthening nurse empathy and responsiveness to the patient as customer. Sound familiar? Aware of unrest among hospital nurses, we decided that, in times like these, simply pressing nurses to give more to the customer would be an affront. Therefore, in tandem with our Medical Center's Nursing Service Department, we launched an exhaustive and fascinating planning process involving more than 200 nurses. We conducted think tanks, focus groups, and one-to-one interviews in order to get to the heart of the issues.

One year later (1987), we produced a seminar called HARMONY: Professional Renewal for Nurses. This one-day seminar has been attended by more than 2,000 nurses across the country. It has been enormously successful—nurses love it and praise it highly. However, it was our feeling that an express route was needed to reach even more nurses. That's how this book came about.

We hope that this book acknowledges and appreciates how hard nurses are working; it is also meant to demonstrate what you as a nurse can *choose* to do in order to accomplish the following:

- Keep or restore your balance and equilibrium.
- Recharge your optimism and enthusiasm.
- Retain or regain your sense of health and well-being.
- Rediscover your commitment to the people you help.
- Renew your vitality and energy.
- Reawaken the satisfaction and fulfillment inherent in caring for people.

We believe in the Professional Renewal concept, its principles and its potential. We hope you will, too.

How to Get the Most from This Book

This book is a self-help course on achieving satisfaction, fulfillment, and a solid sense of accomplishment, as well as greater happiness, as a nurse. Each chapter contains three kinds of material to make your journey through these pages enjoyable, easy, and engaging:

1. **Principles and theory.** The basic principles and theory behind this Professional Renewal concept are explained.
2. **Experiences.** You'll find self-discovery experiences throughout that awaken you and self-help exercises that give you practice.
3. **How-to.** How-to materials present practical ideas, skills, and techniques to help you integrate into your life what you've learned from this book.

Use the book to experience yourself in new and expanded ways. This is a book of experiential learning. It presupposes that the most effective learning is learning in which you are actively involved. Professional Renewal is about experimenting and trying on new thoughts, feelings, and behaviors. But you will need to translate these pages to your own real-life experiences—experiences that matter to you. As you go through the book, apply the concepts and examples to yourself in your day-to-day nursing activities.

Absorb the material slowly. Savor it chapter by chapter. If you read the book quickly and never go back to it, it would be like taking a cross-country train ride on an express ticket and, as you whiz by, never really seeing the multitude of places and experiences you might have on a ticket that allowed you to stop and look around. Take your time. Savor your journey.

The Professional Renewal concept presents a host of ideas, concepts, and principles. Select one area at a time to concentrate on. Make a commitment to strengthen that one aspect of yourself, and other changes will automatically follow. More than anything, we want you to relish this book. Discover yourself and your job fulfillment.

Where Do I Go from Here?

First, you have to decide where you are now! The self-appraisal exercise in the appendix (at the back of this book) can help you establish a baseline from which to measure your progress later. Complete it before you read on, so that you can experience more strongly the benefits of later chapters.

A word about where you are now. Awareness and acceptance are interwoven. By uncritically accepting where you are—whether or not it's where you want to be—you are more likely to open yourself to change. If you mentally beat yourself up or criticize or judge yourself for what you should be, you simply block the process of change and growth. You also sap your own energy and erode your self-esteem. Instead, accept yourself. Acknowledge that where you are is fine. It's where you're supposed to be right now! Because you're there now doesn't mean that you'll be there forever. You have the power of choice!

A Final Word

As authors of this book, we care deeply about nurses and the nursing profession. We wrote this book because we want to share with you our approach to Professional Renewal. We know it works. But it's a no-nonsense approach to improving your life, professionally and personally, and at times we may seem "hard-nosed." If all the care and support we feel for you does not come through every time, we apologize for that up front. We hope you'll charge ahead with us.

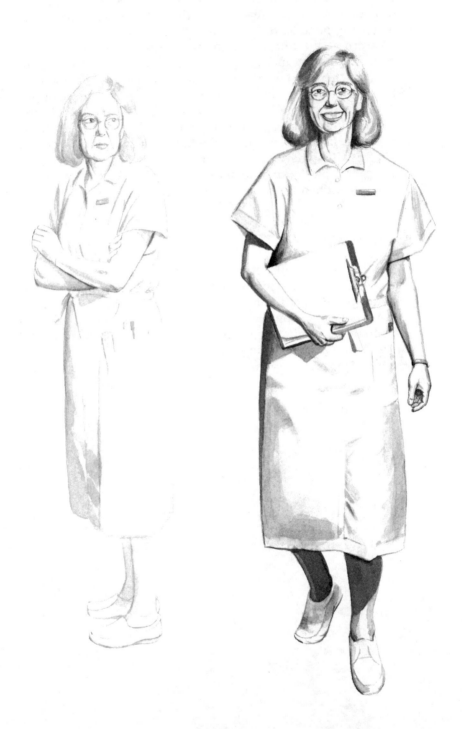

Chapter 1

Taking Charge

Have you ever asked yourself the following questions:

- Why do I fall into the trap of feeling negative at work so often?
- Why do I continue to do the same things over and over when they only make me unhappy and miserable?
- Why can't I feel more on top of my job instead of buried under?

You can answer these questions by taking a hard look at what you're doing that gets you caught in what we call the Self-Defeating Zone and what you can do to get out and stay out:

Self-Defeating Zone

Frustrated	Tense	Resentful
Overwhelmed	Angry	Guilty
Exhausted	Helpless	Short-tempered
Powerless		Anxious

Most hospital nurses report the feelings listed above; they also share many of the struggles listed below:

- ☐ Never-ending demands
- ☐ Intense pace
- ☐ Torn between paperwork and patient care
- ☐ Angry and frustrated about poor staffing
- ☐ Distressed by the scarcity of support services

☐ Upset about supply shortages when you need supplies
☐ Disillusioned about not having enough time to give quality care
☐ Physically tired and emotionally exhausted
☐ Disturbed about having little energy for family and friends

Which feelings do you have, and which struggles do you face?

The Inner Action Model

In this section, we consider the power of the mind. There are different schools of thought about how people change. Some theories postulate that feelings begin the cycle, affecting thoughts and behaviors. Other theories maintain that a person's thoughts begin the cycle—if you can change your thoughts, your feelings and behavior will change. The latter suggests that first you think; these thoughts then trigger feelings; your feelings then influence the actions you take, which in turn produce results. If you learn to take more control of your thoughts, you can increase control of your emotions, actions, and results. This is the essence of the Inner Action Model.

To get a feel for the flow of the Inner Action Model, consider this example:

What are your thoughts about math?

- It's hard.
- I don't like it.
- I'm not good at it.
- I'm average in math skills.
- I love it.
- I hate it.

Let's pursue the example assuming that your original thought was, "I'm not good at math." Let's say that you're getting ready to take your SATs, and these are your thoughts about the math section: "I'll never be able to do it . . . I'm the biggest dunce."

What would you expect your feelings to be as the test day arrives?

☐ Scared
☐ Anxious
☐ Frustrated
☐ Nervous

☐ Panic-stricken
☐ Intimidated
☐ All of the above

Now the test day is here. As you trace the Inner Action cycle, what would you expect your actions to be?

☐ Get stuck on questions; your mind goes blank
☐ Jump from question to question
☐ Change your answer
☐ Tear up your paper; start crying
☐ Give up
☐ Walk out
☐ All of the above

Now you're waiting for your SAT scores to arrive. The mail comes. What results would you expect? Failure or a low score. Then you say, "See, I knew I wasn't good at math." Now you've reinforced or further internalized your original thoughts: "I'm not good at math; I can't do it!"

Thoughts

We are constantly thinking, often without conscious awareness of the choices we have. Our minds are like computers with a lifetime tape packed full of thoughts or "self-talk"—some extremely helpful and enabling, others disabling and severely damaging. Learning to take charge of yourself might involve a whole new process of taking charge of your thoughts.

Wayne Dyer, in *Your Erroneous Zones* (1976, p. 11), says:

You have the power to think whatever you choose to allow into your head. You choose to put it there although you may not know why. You still have the power to make it go away and, therefore, control your mental world. . . . You alone control what enters your head as a thought. If you don't believe this, just ask yourself this question: "If I don't control my thoughts, who does?"

You need to take charge of your thinking and recognize that your thoughts are your own to ponder, to hold, to change, or to bury. To regain control over your thoughts, first stop and listen. Consider your thoughts and the subsequent effects they have upon you. That's the first major premise of Taking Charge: *You control your own thoughts.*

Now let's consider feelings, the next stage in the Inner Action cycle.

Feelings

So far we've established that every feeling is preceded by a thought. Feelings do not just come upon us—they are the direct result of our thinking. Through many years of conditioning, we have programmed ourselves to feel emotions almost simultaneously with our thoughts. These feelings happen so automatically that we've grown unaware of the thought process that triggers them. We end up in a whirlpool of emotions, not knowing how we got there.

In order to take charge of your feelings, you literally need to reprogram or rewire the thinking-feeling link. The way to control your feelings is to address the thoughts that precede them. Feelings, therefore, are choices rather than conditions of life.

What you think is what you feel. The reverse is true as well (that is, what you feel is what you think). Inner harmony involves learning to feel what you *choose* to feel. No doctor can make you feel stupid unless you allow yourself to feel stupid. No hospital policy can cause you to be angry unless you permit yourself to be angry. No coworker can make you sick unless you choose to make yourself think in those terms.

This may be a radical change in the way you are used to thinking. Most of us have grown up in a culture that conditions us to believe that we're not in control of our feelings. Read these statements and see if they sound familiar. Then, look at the transformation this approach instills:

Before Renewal	After Renewal
She makes me angry.	I allowed myself to get mad about what she said.
I can't control my temper.	I can control my temper, but I decided to let them know just how upset I was.
Those minor annoyances from patients really get to me.	I've decided not to let those minor annoyances from patients get to me.
The staffing situation is ruining my health.	I'm letting the staffing situation get to me, and I'm allowing it to affect my health.

Do you recognize the difference? You may be asking, "If it's so simple, why did it take so many years for me to catch on?" Besides cultural conditioning, two other reasons come into play:

1. To be in charge of your thoughts and feelings means taking responsibility for yourself. And frankly, **taking responsibility for yourself is work.** It also means you have to stop blaming others, and that's not as much fun.
2. There are **certain payoffs from the old way of thinking and feeling.** You've probably heard the expression, "You must be getting something from it, otherwise you'd stop doing it." That's a matter only you can deal with.

What are you getting from lingering in the Self-Defeating Zone?

☐ Acknowledgment for how hard I'm working

☐ Pity for how demanding and tough my job is

☐ Safety in that I can hang on to my usual response . . . it's so familiar!

☐ A way to cope . . . even if it's dysfunctional

☐ No need to confront myself with the need to change

☐ Energetic camaraderie that revolves around complaining and commiserating

☐ An endless topic of conversation, without which I might have little left to say

The Point: You might benefit from staying in the Self-Defeating Zone. Many people have grown comfortably miserable there. But are you ready to climb out? Are you sick and tired of being sick and tired? New thinking and new feelings are only a choice away.

Actions

Your thoughts program your feelings. Then your feelings program your actions. Think of yourself as a puppeteer in relation to your own thoughts and feelings. Pulling your own strings is what it comes down to.

Let's look at two examples:

Example 1   Thought: I can't get along with this person . . . it's impossible.
             Feeling: Frustration, anger.
             Action: Slam the phone down.

Example 2   Thought: I'll never be able to take care of all these
                         patients. I know I'm going to forget
                         something.
               Feeling: Being overwhelmed, feeling out of control.
               Action: Medication error.

You're in charge of your actions. No one makes you slam down
the phone. No one else is to blame for your medication error. Let's
explore some examples in depth.

Example 1: Nurse and Difficult Doctor

Background: You, Nurse A, have been told about Dr. Pain-in-the-
             Neck. He's vicious. He has no respect for nurses.
             He will embarrass you in front of others. You need
             to speak with this doctor about your patient, who
             is overmedicated. You need to persuade the physi-
             cian to change the patient's regimen.

Your thoughts could focus on:

Yourself: I'm never going to be able to handle him.
Others: He's impossible.
A Situation: I hope he doesn't come on my shift . . . I'll blow
               it for everyone.

What feelings would you be likely to experience?

   ☐ Fear
   ☐ Intimidation
   ☐ Awkwardness
   ☐ Nervousness

What would be your likely actions?

   ☐ Passive and unassertive behavior
   ☐ Stuttering, stumbling over words
   ☐ Poor eye contact
   ☐ Being tongue-tied
   ☐ Backing off

What would be the likely result of your actions?

   ☐ Doctor remains pushy and insensitive
   ☐ Nurse is unable to express concerns
   ☐ Nurse loses self-respect
   ☐ Patient's medication is not adjusted
   ☐ Risk to patient continues

Example 2: Nurse and Demanding Patient

Background: You, as the second-shift nurse, receive word that your rich patient in Room 301 has been troublesome all day, has been on the call bell frequently, has made unreasonable demands, has complained about care, has been hostile, and so forth.

Your thoughts could focus on:

Yourself: I don't have the patience to deal with this lady.
Others: Rich people think that they're entitled to preferential treatment.
A Situation: I always seem to get the difficult patients.

What feelings would you be likely to experience?

   ☐ Impatience
   ☐ Frustration
   ☐ Guardedness
   ☐ Defensiveness

What do you think your actions would be?

   ☐ Treat the patient in a cold, abrupt manner
   ☐ Do not listen
   ☐ Show little empathy
   ☐ Give orders and commands

What would be the likely result of your actions?

   ☐ Patient continues to be demanding and hostile
   ☐ Patient rings the call bell continuously

Breaking the Cycle

Let's look back on both examples:

- Example 1: Nurse and Difficult Doctor
- Example 2: Nurse and Demanding Patient

In both examples, the nurse ended up in the Self-Defeating Zone, getting poor results. Using the Inner Action Model, let's look at:

1. How to get out of the Self-Defeating Zone
2. How to get more successful results

There are two likely places to *break* the Inner Action cycle to avoid the Self-Defeating Zone and to achieve more successful results:

1. Between thoughts and feelings
2. Between actions and results

Breaking the Cycle between Thoughts and Feelings

You can change or reframe your thoughts. The following examples illustrate how to do this:

Example 1: Nurse and Difficult Doctor

Old Thought	New Thought
I'm never going to be able to handle him.	I can handle him if I stay calm and use my skills.

Old Feelings	New Feelings
Anxiety. Fear.	Confidence. Strength.

Old Action	New Action
Be passive or unassertive. Be tongue-tied.	Speak directly. Express concern and wants.

Old Results	New Results
Doctor is more difficult. Patient medication is not adjusted.	Doctor is more cooperative. Patient medication is adjusted.

Example 2: Nurse and Demanding Patient

Old Thought	New Thought
Rich people think that they deserve preferential treatment.	Rich people are scared when they're sick, too, and sometimes have a harder time letting down their masks.

Old Feelings	New Feelings
Impatience.	Openness.
Defensiveness.	Patience.

Old Action	New Action
Treat the patient in a cold, abrupt manner.	Treat the patient in a warm, friendly way. Listen with understanding.

Old Results	New Results
Patient is more demanding; rings the call bell continuously.	Patient is calmer, more cooperative; rings the call bell less often.

Again, do you see how one thought has the power to set the whole cycle into motion?

Breaking the Cycle between Actions and Results

In the preceding examples, you've seen how to break the Inner Action cycle between thoughts and feelings. Now, let's see how to break the cycle between the actions and the results.

Suppose you choose not to change your thought (that is, "This doctor is a creep"). How could you change your action? What are your options? What could you do differently in order to get your desired results?

Example 1: Nurse and Difficult Doctor

- ☐ Call the physician's office ahead of time and let him or her know that you have concerns about the patient's medication and would like to discuss them when the doctor comes to the floor.
- ☐ Leave a note on the front of the patient's chart documenting patient's symptoms or behavior.
- ☐ Call the physician aside and make a special point of relaying your concerns.
- ☐ Speak right up; get to the point; use a very assertive approach.
- ☐ Do you have additional ideas?

Consider example 2 on the next page; suppose that once again you choose not to change your thoughts. You meet the patient, and you perceive her as a rich, spoiled person. How can you change your actions so that you can achieve more desirable and successful results?

Example 2: Nurse and Demanding Patient

☐ Go into the room and smile; call the patient by name. Listen and empathize with her concerns.

☐ Give lots of reassurance and support.

☐ Express confidence in the patient. Invite her to work with you so that you can help her feel better.

☐ Make an effort to find out what interests the patient, so that you can establish a winning rapport.

☐ Get a volunteer to spend some extra time visiting her.

☐ Invite a patient rep or social worker to offer additional support and services.

☐ Do you have additional ideas?

Let's recap the two main messages inherent in the Inner Action Model:

1. **You have choices.** You can decide how to think, feel, and act to get the results you want.
2. **You are responsible.** It's up to you to take care of your own well-being—personally and professionally. Only you can improve your lot or make yourself happy. It's up to you to take control of your own mind, and then take charge of your feelings and behave in ways that you choose—ways that yield the *results* you want.

Skills and Exercises for Taking Charge

Here are practical tips and techniques to help you integrate the principles of the Inner Action Model.

Observation

New thinking begins with an awareness of old thinking. First, you simply need to observe and tune into your current thinking. When you experience a self-defeating feeling, backtrack. Check out what you were thinking. Note how your thoughts triggered the debilitating feeling. So to begin with, don't set out to change before you've spent time observing yourself. Awareness is 80 percent of a successful change process.

Catch Yourself

When you find yourself saying things such as, "She drives me crazy," or "This job is giving me an ulcer," turn the spotlight on yourself and remind yourself what you are thinking about and how you are behaving at the moment you're doing it. Because it is often difficult to achieve the necessary objectivity, ask a friend to listen to you and point out which statement triggered the self-defeating feeling. Practice rearranging these statements so that you can get yourself back in the driver's seat.

Nip It in the Bud

When you start to fall into the Self-Defeating Zone as a result of your thoughts, feelings, or actions, follow the steps below:

1. Visualize a huge *stop* sign in your mind.
2. Move quickly to envision a glaring neon sign that flashes *choice.*
3. Proceed immediately to back out of the disabling road and drive down the enabling road.

Weed Your Garden

Picture in your mind's eye a big garden overgrown with weeds. The weeds are your self-defeating thoughts, disabling feelings, and debilitating actions. Pull these weeds out by the root and keep pulling them. Kill them off once and for all. Now, plant flowers and vines, that is, empowering thoughts, enabling feelings, and assertive actions.

Cookie Jar of Positive Self-Statements

Write down some positive self-statements on cards. Put these in a jar. Reach in and pull one out in times of high anxiety and self-doubt, as part of your everyday routine. If you wake up not feeling so great, stick a few cards in your uniform pocket and pull them out from time to time during the day.

Here are examples of positive self-statements:

- People tell me I'm unique and special. I just need to believe in myself.
- I have the ability to handle anything I want to handle.
- When you get right down to it, I'm a "winner."

- I've been in rough waters before and came through. I can do it again this time.
- I'm a bright, capable, loving nurse, joyfully giving care to my patients.

"Glad to Be Me" Card File

Get a pack of three-by-five-inch cards and an old recipe file box. On each card, write something you like about yourself . . . something that you value or appreciate about yourself . . . something you're proud of. File headings can include Talents, Skills, Abilities, Accomplishments, Blessings, Attributes, and What Others Tell Me about Me.

For maximum effectiveness, go through your card file two or three times a week. If you're hard-pressed to fill out these cards (your perceptions may be temporarily narrowed), ask a family member or a friend to suggest things you might have overlooked or have been unwilling to admit to yourself. As you think of additional self-enhancing items, write them down and file them. Read your "Glad to Be Me" cards daily to give yourself perspective and strength.

Unstick the Record That's Stuck

You may have fallen into a pattern of excessive replays of negative past events. You're caught in a groove, like the needle on an old record that's worn through. In the midst of trying circumstances and hard times, self-doubts and self-criticism resurface. Remember, you are not forced to pay attention to those persistent little internal voices that create pain or cause you to feel less than competent or lovable. Picture yourself kicking the record needle out of the old, worn-through groove into another groove. Get off of it. Turn off the disabling voices of the past. Introduce new positive and supportive messages. If you refuse to listen to the "old" and dismiss it when it enters your mind, you'll be amazed at how completely it disappears.

Call a Halt to Irrational Thinking

When you're upset or distressed, it's easy to fall into several irrational traps that magnify your anxiety and set in motion a debilitating cycle that ends in poor results. Grab onto your irrational thinking tendencies and put a stop to them:

- **Do you "catastrophize"?** Do you think, "What a disaster! I'll never be able to fix it," or "This is the worse thing that could have happened," or "I'm in a panic, and there's no hope"? When things go wrong, we lose our perspective and exaggerate in our own minds all the most negative, remote possibilities. This tendency prevents us from considering the event in reasonable terms. Make a decision to stop. It's that simple.

- **Do you suffer from "Can't Stand It-itis"?** There's no faster route to driving yourself crazy than to keep insisting that if something doesn't change, you'll go mad. What if it doesn't change? By contracting "Can't Stand It-itis," you block yourself from recognizing the real options you have for coping with difficult situations. Give it up. You'll be glad you did.
- **Are you suffering from "There's No Other Way" paralysis?** This occurs when we attach ourselves to only one way of doing things. We lock into one unworkable solution. This sounds like: "It's impossible! There's absolutely no other way out," or "This is going to ruin my entire day. My hands are completely tied. I can't go another step." Talk about immobilizing messages! Do you hear the stubborn refusal to solve a problem creatively? Let go. Recognize that it may not be the perfect solution or the one you hoped for, but remember that there are always possible solutions.

Become an Experimenter

Often, when people experience the same unsatisfying results, they immediately respond to the question, "What have you tried?" by answering, "Everything!" But, in reality, 8 out of 10 people have tried only one remedy over and over again. In essence, they've tried one thing 100 times.

What is needed are new behaviors . . . a new action strategy. What you've been doing hasn't been working, so how great is the risk of experimenting with a new approach? What possible harm could there be in trying a new way? Unglue yourself and be a person committed to new actions. Doing is action . . . achievement is successful action. Test new possibilities:

- If you've been shut down . . . open up.
- If you've been talking and arguing . . . try listening.
- If you've been passive . . . try being assertive.
- If you've been disorganized . . . try disciplining yourself and organizing what needs to be organized.
- If you've been short and abrupt . . . try a show of patience and understanding.
- If you've felt inadequate . . . enroll in a refresher course on a clinical procedure that you're rusty on.

Get Determined and Go for It

Taking charge of yourself involves more than simply substituting positive thoughts for negative thoughts. It requires a commitment and a determination to be happy and to challenge and wipe out your disabling thoughts, feelings, and actions. If you really want to be in harmony and in control of your own choices, you need to apply diligence and commitment to replacing self-defeating ways with actions that are more self-enhancing and self-advancing.

Start Using Affirmations

Affirmations are self-strengthening statements that you say frequently and repeatedly to yourself as a daily ritual over an extended period of time.

Our minds are like minicomputers . . . constantly recording and storing everything we think and say. Affirmations are those messages you select that you would like to program into your consciousness for the purpose of establishing a new mind-set or supporting yourself in making desired behavioral changes. Make your affirmations short and simple and say them repeatedly, either in your mind or out loud. You can post them on the bathroom mirror or hang them on the refrigerator. Good times to recite your affirmations are at the beginning of the day, while you drive to work, while you're waiting for the elevator, and before you go to sleep. It has been said that it takes 39 days to break a habit and 39 days to make a new one, so be sure to recite your affirmations daily.

You can make up your own affirmations—they tend to work the best—or you can adapt one of the following:

- I am in charge of my thinking.
- I choose only positive feelings for myself.
- I am a person of action.

Do What Works for You

People break the Inner Action cycle differently. For some people, success comes from changing their thinking first. Others experience more success by tackling their actions first. They'll change their actions, which will, in turn, change their attitudes and thoughts. So, for example, if my belief is, "I'm not good at balancing my checkbook," I could change the thought around, or I could change the action (that is, methodically write down the check number, date, purpose and amount of the check, and add and subtract accordingly). After I experience success, I will be able to go back and think differently—that is, "When I take the time, I can keep a balanced checkbook." Decide what works for you and do it.

Summary

In this chapter, we've introduced the Inner Action Model and demonstrated how feelings, actions, and results all follow from your thoughts. Taking charge of your thoughts is the first step toward controlling your feelings and directing your actions for positive results. That means getting out and staying out of the Self-Defeating Zone.

The exercises in this chapter have been designed to enable you to tune in to your current thought patterns, identify where they are defeating you, and turn them to positive advantage. Remember, practice will make that second nature.

So, take charge today! And stay out of that Self-Defeating Zone! Turn those negatives into positives—now and for your wonderful future!

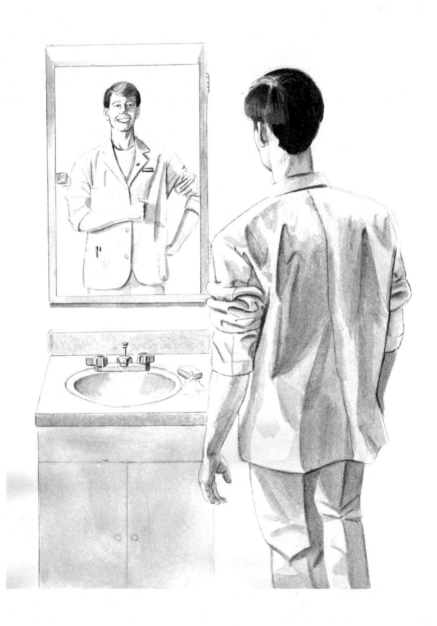

Chapter 2

Your Relationship with Yourself

Are you happy being a nurse? Would your response sound something like this:

> How can anyone be happy being a nurse, considering the conditions we have to put up with? Long hours, poor pay, backbreaking labor, constant staffing shortages, an avalanche of paperwork, tremendous responsibility with little power, inadequate support services, incredible demands, with little respect and appreciation. Give me a break!

If your response is similar, there is a good chance you've gone too far in giving up control over your own happiness. This happens when you see unhappiness as caused entirely by external circumstances—when you fail to see your own choice in the matter.

But you can work to shift that outlook to a happier, more content frame of mind by becoming a more *internally controlled person.* After all, if you insist that the hospital, your nursing management, or the medical bureaucracy is responsible for the way you feel, you've put yourself in the position of waiting until they decide to change before you can feel better. That doesn't make much sense, does it? And besides, you may have a long wait.

Being happy as a nurse is not a complex affair. It involves living and working in an emotional world controlled by you, not by others. Only you can create your own happiness. You are the conductor of your own internal harmony.

As Dr. Wayne Dyer wrote in *The Sky's the Limit,* published in 1983 by Simon and Schuster (p. 243), "There is no way out of the

17

box of externally caused unhappiness that you can open for yourself other than through the internal route."

During the course of our travels, we have listened to many nurses
and have heard over and over about their search for peace and a
sense of inner completion. For many of you, especially in difficult
times, nursing is a path full of pitfalls on which you may have lost
your footing.

If this applies to you, you need to regain your footing on the path
toward happiness and compassion by dealing with the present, not
the future. You may be postponing happiness until a time when
staffing is full, when your reporting relationship changes, when the
order-entry system is up and running, or when some other
hypothetical change occurs in your external environment. If this
is what you're waiting for in order to be happy, you may be chasing
an illusion that will never come to pass. Consider this short fable:

> A big cat saw a little cat chasing its tail and asked, "Why are
> you chasing your tail so?" Said the kitten, "I have learned that
> the best thing for a cat is happiness, and that happiness is my
> tail. Therefore, I am chasing it, and when I catch it, I shall have
> happiness."
>
> Said the old cat, "My son, I, too, have paid attention to the
> problems of the universe. I, too, have judged that happiness is
> in my tail. But, I have noticed that whenever I chase after it, it
> keeps running away from me, and when I go about my busi-
> ness, it just seems to come after me wherever I go."

The Time Is Now

There is only one moment in which you can experience happiness,
and that moment is now. Taking charge of the present is essential
to creating your happiness. To accomplish this, however, you have
to decide to *choose* happiness. Your ability to choose happiness for
yourself in every moment depends on a positive self-concept and
the art of self-love.

The Concept: Loving yourself means accepting yourself as you
are right now.

In *Living with Joy* (p. 43), published by H. J. Kramer, Tiburon,
California, 1986, Sanaya Roman explains this concept further:

> There are no exceptions to the contract; it is an agreement with
> yourself to appreciate, validate, accept and support who you are
> at this moment. It means living in the present time. Many of

you look back into the past with regret, thinking of how you could have handled a situation in a higher way, imagining if only you had done this or that, things would have worked out better. Some of you look into the future to make who you are right now inadequate. The past can assist you if you remember the times in which you succeeded in creating positive memories and the future can be your friend if you see that in picturing it you are creating a vision of the next step. Do not make yourself wrong because you have not yet achieved it. It is important to love who you are now without reservation.

Who Am I?

Answer this question, and you've taken the first step toward achieving a positive self-image. Your answer may well reflect the expectations that others impose upon you—what others tell you that you should be, what you must do, how you should behave. All of these family and societal expectations that you've taken on can be major obstacles to your self-love. In the following passage, which is reprinted from "A Poet's Advice to Students" in *A Miscellany*, published by Harcourt Brace Jovanovich, Inc., e e cummings portrays the power of this all-too-human condition:

> To be nobody—but yourself—in a world that is doing its best, night and day, to make you everybody else—means to fight the hardest battle which any human being can fight and never stop fighting.

It's tempting—and very easy—to grant others authority over what you should do and what's good for you. This inclination is largely a legacy from childhood. Your own self-image may still be determined by early events when you experienced hurt, failure, and humiliation. It could still contain the perceptions of a demanding teacher, a domineering friend, or a critical parent. The judgments of these people were crucial to your developing self-concept.

Although it is true that your earliest impressions of yourself were made by the opinions of others, it is not true that you need to carry these impressions around with you forever. It's time that you discarded these old self-images. They no longer fit, and, chances are, they work against you. It's time that you replaced them with new self-images that reflect who you are today—self-images that work for you.

Take a good look at everything you've been told about yourself, and ask yourself some key questions:

1. Does this view of myself really *fit* where I want to be?
2. Does it bring me happiness and joy?
3. Does this self-concept make me feel good?

Ultimately, it's your own experience that counts. Your own experience keeps you on the path toward happiness. This requires a constant sorting out of self-concepts, picking through and consciously deciding which aspects of your self-image to keep as relevant and positive, and which to discard as outdated and destructive.

The Concept: Do more of what works in your life and less of what doesn't.

If that means shedding old shackles and wiping the slate clean, then what are you waiting for? Take your mental eraser and wipe away limiting self-concepts of the past. Choose to make self-respecting new images that release you and give you new freedom.

Will the Real Me Please Stand Up?

You actually have many self-images. You have self-images regarding your physical, intellectual, social, and emotional selves. You have self-images about your special abilities—such as music, art, athletics, auto mechanics, academics, and so forth. You may have a strong professional self-image as a nurse. And whether your overall self-appraisal is positive or negative may vary from day to day, even from moment to moment. However, beneath all these self-images is a *core* that is who you are, and that *core* is your own irreducible self-worth.

Think of your *core* self-worth as the deepest inner roots connecting you with yourself. Your *core* self-worth is determined by you. It is not dependent on the opinion of others. It's entirely up to you what sense of self-worth you choose. It's only a question of "Are you for yourself, or are you against yourself?"

Nurses often are their own worst enemies. If you want to be your own best friend, you'll need to construct a solid, positive concept of your own self-worth. That self-worthiness becomes a constant—a given—and has nothing to do with your day-to-day feelings and behaviors. You may not like your own behavior from time to time, but that won't shake your *core* concept of self-worth.

Imagine your individual self-images, feelings, and behaviors as branches of your tree of life. Your branches may shake during a windy, emotional storm, but your roots—that is, your self-worth—never give way. They are deeply planted and completely insulated. And your day-to-day assessments of yourself should not alter your perception of your intrinsic self-worth. You are much more than the sum of your feelings and behaviors at any particular moment. You may not be pleased with your performance with Dr. X, but that doesn't mean you are without worth. Once you choose an unshakable sense of self-worth, you create a regulating device for all the times when it's necessary to keep your balance.

Simple, Not Easy

Keeping a strong sense of self-worth is a simple concept, but it is easier said than done. A bad day, a couple of demanding patients, and a bout with one egotistic doctor—and your whole sense of self-worth may deflate like a balloon too weak to pop. As a nurse, one of your greatest challenges is to keep your balance no matter what comes along. When someone is pulling on you, when another is calling you, and a third is demanding something of you, instead of blowing a fuse, plug in to your center of self-worth. Connect with all those important and valuable assets that make up your positive self-image. Think of people who walk tightropes with the greatest of ease—their unshakable self-worth makes that possible. And yours can do the same for you.

I'm Me, Not You

One way to love yourself more is to stop comparing yourself with others. When you're in the business of comparing, you're telling your subconscious, "Who I am isn't good enough." This leads to an internal dialogue of self-criticism that eats away at your self-esteem.

Do you constantly compare yourself with your colleagues and others? Are these comparisons likely to be unfavorable to yourself? "She's smarter. He's so together. She knows exactly what to say and how to say it." This kind of thinking creates a dull pain deep down that drains your self-esteem and, with it, your energy. If you habitually compare yourself unfavorably with others, you may no longer even be conscious that you're doing it. But you probably are aware that you feel "blah."

It's time to stop comparing yourself with others and start collecting all your life experiences so that you can regard them as the substance of what you were born to be about. Whether you label them good or bad, right or wrong, these experiences make up your total being to the present moment.

You're unique. Admit it. Respect your uniqueness, and you're on the way to self-love. This process of self-acceptance allows you to stop comparing yourself unfavorably with others and emphasizes that you're one-of-a-kind.

What's at the Bottom of It?

Talking with many nurses, we learned the importance of a positive self-concept in determining nursing success and satisfaction. One nurse summed it up this way, "It all depends on how I feel about myself on any given day. If I feel good about me, I can handle just about anything."

Self-acceptance is critical to your sense of self-worth. Self-acceptance means liking the entire you and taking pleasure in being you. By denying any part of you, you're denying yourself. The only way you're going to feel whole and satisfied is to embrace all of you.

Do you accept yourself 100 percent? Or is your answer a "Yes, but . . . ," followed by a trail of qualifiers? Do you view yourself as physically unattractive? Are there things about yourself that you hate? Do self-appraisals include criticisms such as "My nose is too big," "I'm too fat," "I'm uncomfortable socially," "I'm afraid to try anything new," and so forth? Do you accept yourself as a capable, intelligent person? Or do you feel stupid, dull, and incompetent? Is your inner dialogue belittling? "Sure, I did okay in nursing school, *but* really, I'm not very smart," or, "If I went to another unit, I wouldn't know which end was up."

Your inadequate self-image may actually reflect a mistaken understanding of the meaning of intelligence. The concept of intelligence is fascinating but often misunderstood. Dr. Wayne Dyer describes aptitude as a function of time rather than as some inborn quality. In fact, he says that the happier you make yourself, the more intelligent you are. If we devote enough practice and time, we each have the capacity to be proficient at almost anything. Dyer believes that we choose to exercise our intelligence in various select areas, and that these are the areas in which we excel.

Stop and think about all the subject areas in which you choose not to use your brain power. Now review the list in your mind and consider the negative results you achieve in these areas. If you're weighted down with old, negative messages, it may be time to revamp your view of your own aptitude and how you choose to use it.

Perfectly Imperfect

Self-acceptance also means accepting that you're perfectly imperfect. Can you forgive yourself for past mistakes and let them go once and for all? Forgiving yourself frees you from the inner chains that you've allowed to imprison you. Forgiving yourself gives way to self-acceptance, and self-acceptance is the key to forgiving yourself.

We all have secrets deep within us, our own awareness of our own imperfections. What are some of the secrets you hold deep inside? The way to know if you need to engage in forgiving yourself is to resurrect these secrets. If there's still negative emotional energy associated with them, then release them. Let go and forgive yourself.

Shred and Flush

To rid yourself of your secrets, try this little ceremony. Take pieces of note paper and write down all the burdensome secrets you feel guilty about or bothered by, one to each piece of paper. Find a deep container and prepare for your shredding ceremony. After you've written down all the secrets, begin to shred them one by one into tiny pieces until all you're looking at is a pile of scraps. Take this residue and flush it down the toilet, saying "Goodbye!" once and for all. Say to yourself, or out loud, "I am forgiving and releasing myself from these secrets! I am free!" And believe it!

Don't allow those secrets back into your psyche again. If the thoughts do recur, let them pass right through you. Immediately say to yourself, "I have forgiven and released myself from this secret! I am free!" Visualize the shredding and flushing ceremony, and breathe a sigh of release!

But I Have Flaws!

Self-acceptance requires coming to terms with your limitations. Everyone has limitations. Let's talk about the parts of you that are not so great. Let's call these parts your limitations. These are the characteristics that can ruin your life if you allow them to. Of course, the choice is yours. These limiting characteristics affect your self-concept and, in turn, your thoughts and actions. One limiting characteristic may be your need to be perfect or right all the time. Or, it may be the angry, resentful, hurt sides of you, or the part of you that feels ugly, unworthy, or unforgiving. This is the stuff we beat ourselves up with day after day. Limiting characteristics can keep you stuck in cycles of unhappiness, self-doubt, pain, and misery.

So how do you handle these limitations? First, imagine placing your limiting characteristics under a magnifying glass and magnifying them all out of proportion. Become totally aware of how they work against you. Once they're exaggerated, you're ready to recognize them at every turn.

Meanwhile, build up those enabling characteristics that supersede your limiting characteristics. For example, if your limiting characteristic is resentment, then your enabling characteristic needs to be forgiveness. If your limiting characteristic is sadness, your enabling characteristic is the capacity for joy. If your limiting characteristic is being judgmental, your enabling characteristic needs to be tolerance and love. Get the idea? So, instead of saying, "I'm a resentful, sad, judging person," say, "I'm a forgiving, joyful, accepting, and loving person."

The Concept: What you focus on is what you get.

It's important for you to recognize your ability to change your focus—and to remember that you already have the qualities you wish you had. All of these qualities are already in your repertoire. You need only amplify them and give them prominence. You can do this if you pay attention to them and stop paying attention to your limitations. Limitations are like the class bully—if you give in to them, they'll always be hanging around to bother you. But if you ignore them, eventually they'll go away. As Sanaya Roman writes in *Living with Joy* (p. 69):

> It's important to become aware of the attention you pay to who you are not. You may say: "I need to do this or that. Why am I always so unorganized, so unfocused?" Be aware that as you think of your lack of certain qualities, you bring that lack into yourself. Whatever you pay attention to is what you create. The more you see within yourself when you want to become, the more you will become it.

An Identity Crisis in the World of Nursing

This chapter has focused on your internal world and your relationship with yourself. As an individual nurse, however, you must recognize that you exist in a professional world that is in a state of flux and transition. The profession of nursing is in an identity crisis. In an external world that is full of chaos, confusion, and turmoil, it's no wonder that many nurses feel turmoil on the inside. However, beware of allowing yourself to get pulled into the "mob mind-set," which may not reflect your own true feelings and beliefs. Your identity as a nurse may not be in crisis. You may actually be part of a silent majority! The point is, you must be certain you're consciously choosing what you feel, and not simply joining the crowd.

Take Stock of Your Choice of Profession

It's important that you periodically explore your feelings in relation to your choice of the profession of nursing. Trust yourself. Ask yourself, "Is nursing really what I want? Is it bringing happiness and joy into my life? Does nursing continue to provide me with the meaning and purpose I want from my life's work?''

Sometimes, when we're treading water in the pool of discontent and disillusionment, we're afraid to dive down and see what's at the bottom of things. Avoidance is a game many of us play all too well. But the longer we avoid this self-confrontation, the larger the monster of our own creation grows. It goes back to the old saying, ''There's nothing to fear but fear itself.''

If you're having serious doubts about your profession and are submerging these doubts, let them rise to the surface by talking them out with a trusted person who is skilled at listening. Chances are, you need to talk them out and think them through, to confront the fear you've attached to them.

Many nurses discover their real love for the nursing profession only after sorting out the negative external factors and weighing those against their own internal motivations and gratifications. Others discover that they are not sure that nursing is where they want to be. However, they do feel a sense of relief just for having looked at their doubts and not hiding from them. Nurses who are uncertain about their choice of profession need to give themselves the freedom to question and explore this choice without self-judgment and guilt.

Get Off the Fence

Regardless of the outcome, taking stock of your compatibility with and commitment to the profession of nursing brings renewal and refreshment. Indecisiveness, vacillation, sitting on the fence—these drain energy.

Summary

Being your own best friend doesn't always come easily. The relationship you establish with yourself becomes the basis for your happiness. This chapter has spotlighted core issues, such as the importance of accentuating the positives of your life through a serious look at self-worth, self-acceptance, and self-forgiveness. You saw that flaws, imperfections, and limitations are also a part of you and need to be embraced and well-tamed so that they never interfere in your quest to be all you are capable of being.

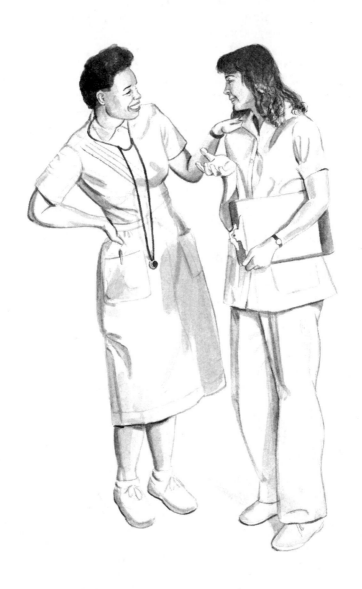

Chapter 3

Your Relationship with Others

Your success and happiness as a nurse really depend on your ability to relate to others in a healthy manner. However, it is not easy to relate harmoniously to all people all of the time. Doing so requires four resources:

- A positive self-image
- Vital inner reserves of self-respect, self-appreciation, and self-confidence
- Positive people skills
- Effective interpersonal skills

Successful work relationships follow a fundamental principle: *The way you treat yourself dictates how others will treat you.* However, no matter how good you feel about yourself, it also takes a wealth of sharpened human relations skills to enable you to feel that you are in charge of your work world.

The following quote from Leo F. Buscaglia's *Loving Each Other* (Fawcett Books, New York City, 1986, p. 167) says it well:

You are at the center of all your relationships, therefore you are responsible for your self-esteem, growth, happiness and fulfillment. Don't expect the other person to bring you these things. You must live as if you are alone and others are the gifts offered to help you enrich your life.

So the theme once again is: Take responsibility. The world of nursing involves difficult and demanding issues in human relationships, and it's more important than ever for nurses to cultivate their own wellsprings of self-respect, self-acceptance, and self-love. Once you're in touch with your own source of love and strength, you won't feel so wounded or hurt when, for example, a doctor treats you with disrespect. If you are balanced and centered in your own power, no systems breakdown at work can throw you off.

We've already discovered that self-talk can be a valuable tool in helping you to keep your balance. Tell yourself that you can keep your balance and center and that you are not dependent on others to feel good, to feel satisfied, and to feel appreciated.

Respect

It's easy to respect yourself when others around you respect you. The true test, however, is to respect yourself when others do not treat you as you would like them to treat you.

The Concept: Surrender any need you have for others to validate you! It's OK to want validation—it's another thing to need it. When only validation from others can make you feel good about yourself, you give away your own power.

Sometimes you'll find yourself around people who do not treat you with the respect you believe that you deserve. Act with calm and dignity, and remember: They probably don't respect themselves. Think of the faces and voices you encounter all day—colleagues, supervisors, doctors, patients, families, support staff, and others. Think of all the times you felt hurt, angry, insulted, offended, and taken for granted. Consider these painful feelings in terms of the words of Sanaya Roman (*Living with Joy,* p. 59), and find a refreshing perspective:

> No matter how good you feel about yourself, there will always be those who do not treat you in a respectful way, for they have not learned how to treat themselves in a loving way. The relationship you have with others can only be as good as the relationships they have with themselves.

This perspective on understanding others' deficits can help you stay off the defensive and keep your inner balance. Instead of personalizing the negative behavior of others as an affront to yourself, you can tip the scales by recognizing that it's their own vulnerabilities that are coming into play.

Your Identity as a Nurse

Maintaining a center in your identity as a nurse is crucial to maintaining your sense of balance. Do you celebrate yourself in your role as a nurse? Or do you berate yourself because anything you do is never good enough? Self-doubt, critical self-judgment, lack of self-respect—these are not the road to joy. Instead, try acceptance, love, and respect for yourself as a nurse. Others cannot give you these things. You are the source of your own good feelings; others are simply your audience. Tune into the energy you put out to other people; for what you put out, most likely, is what you'll get back. Even though the relationship people have with themselves affects how they will relate to you, most often if you convey strength and confidence, others will respect you and trust you; if you demonstrate openness and acceptance, others will do the same for you; and if you radiate honor and appreciation for who you are, others will join you. If you honor the world of others, their time and their values, they will honor yours.

Forgiveness

If you're still hanging on to old differences and past hurts, you're probably experiencing the same anger over and over again. Maybe it's irritation with your boss or a colleague, or maybe it's someone who has let you down along the way. The person you resent may be affected, but they'll never be as affected by this as you are. That's because judgment, resentment, and anger toward others rob you of your own inner acceptance and joy. Every time you hurt others, you are really hurting yourself. That's why forgiveness—of self and of others—is so important. It heals and it frees your own inner source of goodwill and caring.

Handling Human Differences

Accepting that others are not exactly like you is one of the greatest challenges in human relations. Often, the greater the perceived dissimilarity, the greater the struggle becomes. When you encounter someone at work who is different from you, you may unconsciously enter into a power struggle to deal with this difference. Instead, try accepting the other person as he or she is. It really doesn't require much—just extending the kind of respect you'd like to receive.

The nursing arena is full of conflicts, and it is imperative to learn not to be pulled into the negativism often generated by others. When you find yourself in the midst of a power struggle, try this exercise: Call a brief time-out for yourself in your mind. Take a deep breath and decide that you're not going to get caught up in this conflict.

If someone is pushing for a fight, simply choose not to participate; step aside and embrace a deeper level of compassion.

Freedom to be who you are begins by letting go of trying to change others and by giving others freedom to be who they are. That's easier said than done, isn't it? But the truth of the matter is, *it's the only way that works.* By continually focusing on what's wrong with another person, you only drive negativism deeper.

Instead, switch your focus. Bring out the good in others, recognize their inner beauty, and let them know that you value and appreciate them as they are. Before you know it, you'll have provided the basis for a harmonious relationship! Sometimes, it makes sense to tackle the problem head on, in an assertive manner. Other times, it's best to take a diagonal approach—a nonconfrontational, nonthreatening style really can work in a world of human diversity. As Sanaya Roman suggests in *Living with Joy* (p. 37):

> The more you focus on problems between you, or on what's wrong with other people, the more you will find relationships going downhill. When people first get together they are so focused on the good in each other, it is said they wear rose-colored glasses. This is a great gift to each other, for as each pays attention to the good in the other they help each other create it. Loving people is a commitment to holding a high vision of them even as time and familiarity take their toll.

Taking Risks

Increasing satisfactions and joys at work requires taking risks in your interpersonal relationships. Staying with the safe and familiar can only lead to stagnation and discontent.

Nurses are great at giving. However, openness to receiving friendship and support from others is the second half of the equation. But openness involves risk—risk of vulnerability and risk of relinquishing defensive postures that cut you off from others. It means peeling away the layers of mask that uphold your image of who you think you are. Such masks only keep you isolated from all the good others can bring you—support, comfort, understanding, love, and concern. Being vulnerable does not imply weakness or lack of self-confidence. Instead, it demonstrates a great deal of faith and trust in yourself. Vulnerability says, "I am not perfect. I am a real person with hurt, pain, confusion, and madness. I need to be understood, supported, and comforted. I need you." Vulnerability is the gateway to intimacy and closeness. Without it, relationships drift into emptiness and superficiality. When you take a risk and show the real you, you give others permission to do the same. *Living with Joy* (Sanaya Roman, p. 49) expresses it this way: "One of the greatest gifts you can give others is opening to their love for you."

The Issue of Power

Another major source of conflict for nurses is power. Chances are, you have preconceived notions of "powerful people" whose ruthlessness brings harm to those who fall under their domination. And consciously or unconsciously, you probably have formed a number of negative associations about power and the actions of powerful people. This is unfortunate, because this frame of reference can only hold you back from exercising your own personal power, and you may remain confused about ways to express it.

Let's differentiate between two kinds of power: positional power and personal power. We're used to thinking about positional power in our organizations. Granted, personal power has the formal authority to make decisions and changes. You may not have this "positional power"; however, each of us has a great deal of personal power to influence decisions and make important changes happen. The bottom line is: Choose to use your personal power and use it effectively.

When considering the issues surrounding either kind of power, it is necessary to see the difference between people who only participate in a masquerade of power and people who truly are powerful. Think for a moment about the powerful authority figures in your own life. What is it about those people that you admire? Are you reminded of people who triggered feelings of depreciation, ignored you, or put you down? This is not true power.

True power is expressed by persons with the ability to reach out and encourage others to explore and strive toward their own full potential. True power is motivating, loving, and supporting others. One of the most accurate barometers of true power is this: When you are with someone you perceive as "powerful," do you feel better about yourself, expanded in your being? If, through your contact with this person, you have found an entrance to a deeper level of your being, then you have experienced the true meaning of power. You'll know it, too, because you'll be recharged and revived by the experience. Such powerful—and empowering—people will encourage you to express your own true power more fully.

So, now that you've gained a fresh perspective on power, doesn't it challenge you to reassess the power structure at work? Isn't it interesting how this new perspective deflates some of the pompous egos you have to deal with? And, in the meantime, how it demystifies the acquisition of power? Chances are, you, yourself, have a lot more power than you realize.

Peaceful Coexistence

Believe it or not, peaceful coexistence really is possible in the workplace. To achieve it, first regard all conflict as neutral. Conflict is neutral—unless you assign a meaning to it. But conflict can mean an opportunity for you to grow and to learn. The very people with whom you experience conflict are the people who hold the key to your own healing and learning. Take a risk and get to know them. By knowing them, you'll know yourself. When you find people difficult, chances are that you are viewing a part of yourself that you dislike. Let go of self-judgment, and you will experience less judgment from others. People criticize because they are critical of themselves. Their actions and words are often a statement about their own level of self-doubt. Remain calm and centered, and you can affect those around you positively.

When something happens that would normally make you feel defensive or closed, when you would normally pull away, choosing to feel hurt, you have another choice. If instead you are willing to open your heart just one more notch, experience a little more compassion and understanding for other people, you will find yourself able to send them love and create a feeling of peace for yourself. The following quotation from Sanaya Roman (*Living with Joy,* pp. 115–17) tells how to achieve this peace:

> Right now, make the decision that you can bring inner peace into your life. Make the decision that you're going to open your heart even more, be more compassionate, more understanding, more loving, and more forgiving of everyone you know. Form a picture in your mind of yourself going through the next week, and see yourself coming from a totally new level of peace. See the smile on your face and the joy in your heart.

Summary

Only you can determine the quality of your relationships with others by taking responsibility, by respecting yourself and others, and by recognizing and accepting human differences.

Leo Buscaglia summarizes these principles beautifully in the following 10 excerpts from *Loving Each Other* (pp. 150–67):

- Don't be concerned about what you can get from a relationship. Instead, concern yourself with what you can bring to it.
- Expect what is reasonable, not what is perfect.
- Learn to listen. You don't learn anything from hearing yourself talk.
- Learn to bend. It's better than breaking.
- Don't be afraid of disagreements and arguments. The only people who don't argue are people who don't care or are dead. In fact, don't have short arguments. Make certain they are thoroughly over and done with.
- Don't make the other's problems yours. It only makes solving it twice as difficult.
- Don't brood. Get on with living and loving. You don't have forever.
- Don't hold on to anger, hurt or pain. They steal your energy and keep you from love.
- Don't overanalyze your relationships.
- Remember that a relationship is a pooling of resources. That means that with each relationship you are not only giving, you are becoming more.

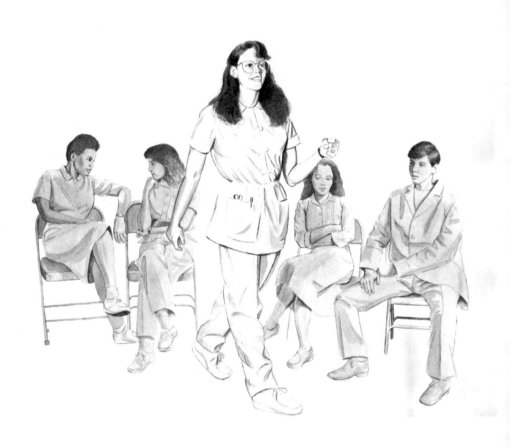

Chapter 4

Assertiveness

If you randomly ask people in any part of the country what they want in life, you'll probably get a lot of different answers. If you push a little harder, dig a little deeper, what many people are saying is, "I want to be happy." For most of us, that means being able to form and keep healthy, positive relationships. What grows in the "garden" of relationships depends on what and how we nourish it.

Reaching a point in your relationships where you feel good about yourself and others and your interactions isn't easy. Success at relationships takes skill and practice—a lot of skill and a lot of practice. In chapter 3, "Your Relationships with Others," we talked about accepting yourself and others, about some problems with competition, and about potentially damaging ways of relating. Putting this knowledge into action with friends and coworkers is harder than gaining insight or reawakening ideals you've had for a while. Although understanding and knowledge are the first ingredients, you need to master some skills to change the way you communicate in order to achieve the quality you desire in relationships. These skills will help you to clearly convey what you think, feel, and want.

The Key Is Practice!

Have you ever watched a child learning to tie a shoe? It can take hours of effort to get the laces to go the right way and stay there. Children have short fuses when they learn; they try for a while and then abandon the new task, only to come back again and again until they master it. As adults, we forget about our childhood frustration, tears, and clenched fists when the bows would mysteriously unravel. As adults, we hardly notice our nimble hands performing a routine daily task. Those hours of trying and retrying are long forgotten.

Acquiring positive human relations skills is even more complex. We have all gone to a party and watched as some people mingle, talking easily with strangers. These people stand out because their ability to relate to people seems effortless. But if you ask them what they do to socialize with people so well, they probably couldn't tell you. Their hours of practice as a child trying out different behaviors are lost from memory. By now, many of their skills are so automatic they are unrecognized.

With both of these examples, acquiring a skill requires persistent effort and reexamining of outcomes. If you want to develop more satisfying relationships with people, first you will need the following:

- To have a real desire to change some of your behavior
- To have a willingness to take some risks, starting with small, fairly safe steps
- To understand that you won't always get what you want, no matter how skilled you become
- To be willing to make a mistake and try again
- To be your own best friend and give yourself rewards and positive feedback
- To use the Inner Action Model (see chapter 1) to stay focused on the results you want
- To tune into your inner dialogue and self-talk
- To find a friend or coworker with whom to practice situations
- To see the gradual changes you have made over time and congratulate yourself on your accomplishments

Behaviors You Can Choose

You can choose to be assertive, nonassertive, or aggressive. These behaviors are described in the following sections, with exercises and examples to help you change and become more assertive.

Assertive Behavior

To get what you want and to feel good about your relationships, you have to stand up for your rights and express your feelings, opinions, and preferences in a way that is honest, direct, and shows respect for others. You will not get the results you want by being unclear about what you want, by backing down at the first hint of refusal, or by giving in to the "much more important" needs of others.

Assertive behavior includes asking for what you want and expressing your feelings in ways that show respect for yourself and for the people you are communicating with.

Assertiveness is:

- Knowing who you are
- Knowing what you want
- Knowing how to get it
- Believing you can get it

Nonassertive Behavior

Nonassertive behavior, or submission, means giving in to others' requests, demands, or feelings without regard to your own wants or feelings. People behave in nonassertive ways because they fear displeasing others, because they fear rejection and retaliation. This passivity is typically intended to please others. But giving in may require you to dismiss your own feelings as unreal or unimportant. This can be very costly, because when you suppress your feelings, they tend to leak out over time in subtle, negative actions that hurt relationships.

If you rely primarily on others for your self-esteem (to give you good feelings about yourself, or rewards for your accomplishments), their disapproval can be very threatening. First of all, you need to be your own best friend and believe in your own worth. You can feel good about yourself and trust that feeling. Secondly, it helps to differentiate between your self-worth and your behavior. Every action or behavior is a tiny expression of yourself. No one is perfect. You may be afraid that somebody won't like something you do or say, but don't confuse that with total rejection. "You can't please all of the people all of the time," anyway, but you can still be a good person. Good people decide to change their behavior because they believe a different course of action will get them what they want, or because they agree with others' disapproval of their past behavior. It's uncomfortable to receive criticism, but it's important not to exaggerate that discomfort into feelings of worthlessness.

Sometimes people are nonassertive because they believe that others will pull away in hurt and anger, or try to get back at them. This is a possibility. But the fear of withdrawal or retaliation is frequently unrealistic, and some objectivity is often enough to put this fear into perspective. In a situation where you're afraid of withdrawal or retaliation, consider these questions:

- Have you been assertive with this person, and did that person respond with rejection or retaliation?

- What is the worst possible thing that could happen if they reacted that way?
- Is that likely to occur?
- What will be the long-term effect on the relationship if you hold your thoughts or feelings inside?
- What does it feel like to live in constant fear of rejection? Is the discomfort worth it? Are you getting anything from the discomfort?

At times, you may consciously choose to behave in nonassertive ways. Your manager might have you work nights if you are direct and disagree with the proposed vacation schedule. Perhaps the manager has retaliated against other staff members who have disagreed with his or her ideas. If you choose to go along with the schedule, you're making an objective decision. You might also decide to look for a position on a unit where the manager is more democratic and open. Or, you may like the people you work with well enough to tolerate the manager's behavior. The point of this example is that your self-worth is not in question, and you have used objective facts to make a rational decision to get what you want.

Aggressive Behavior

It's important to know the difference between aggressive behavior and assertive behavior. Aggressive behavior means standing up for your rights, but expressing yourself in ways that violate the rights of others or that fail to show them respect. Such behaviors may include sarcasm or humiliating insults (also called "killer words") or overpowering the other person in order to win or dominate. Some people react with aggressive behavior when they feel threatened and unsafe. Aggressiveness can also occur when feelings of anger, hurt, and disappointment are allowed to build up over time. When many small hurts accumulate over time, the result is often a "big bang" of disappointment and anger.

People are aggressive in order to protect themselves from threatening situations. The aggressive response becomes automatic, as do the assumptions about the threat. But once again, how realistic is this threat? It is helpful to short-circuit this reaction and recognize the feelings of tension and fear behind it. Tune in to your thoughts and feelings that may be disabling. Take time to check out what's real by using these questions:

- Am I really in danger?
- What rights does the other person have, and do they conflict with mine?

- What can I do to protect myself without becoming aggressive?
- What power do I actually have in this situation?
- What do I want to have happen?
- What are my choices?

It is important to differentiate between irritation and aggression. For example, if you've said that you cannot work a double shift today, and a manager or supervisor repeatedly insists that you do work the extra shift, you might feel pushed and irritated. You can state your feelings without becoming aggressive toward the supervisor: "I am really irritated with your insistence. I said I couldn't work, and I don't want to discuss it further." Anger is a normal reaction in some situations, but it doesn't mean that you automatically have to become aggressive. You can still get what you want without clobbering other people. Figure 4-1 summarizes the difference between assertive, nonassertive, and aggressive behavior.

Figure 4-1. A Comparison of Nonassertive, Assertive, and Aggressive Behavior

	Nonassertive	Assertive	Aggressive
Characteristics of behavior	Does not express wants, ideas, and feelings or expresses them in a self-deprecating way	Expresses wants, ideas, and feelings in direct and appropriate ways	Expresses wants, ideas, and feelings at the expense of others
Your feelings when you act this way	Anxious, disappointed with yourself; often angry and resentful later	Confident, feel good about yourself at the time and later	Self-righteous, superior; sometimes embarrassed later
Other people's feelings about themselves when they act this way	Guilty or superior	Respected, valued	Humiliated, hurt
Other people's feelings about you when you act this way	Irritation, pity, disgust	Usually respect	Angry, vengeful
Outcome	Don't get what you want; anger builds up	Often get what you want	Often get what you want at the expense of others; others feel justified at "getting even"
Payoff	Avoids unpleasant situation; avoids conflict, tension, confrontation	Feels good; respected by others; improved confidence; improved relationships	Vents anger, feels superior

Source: Adapted from Jakubowski, P., and Lange, A. J. *The Assertive Option: Your Rights and Responsibilities,* published by Research Press, copyright 1978, pp. 42–43.

It is important to recognize that no one is totally aggressive, assertive, or submissive. The major point is to make a conscious choice about the type of behavior you want to use—to be in control of your actions and reactions.

Exercise

Let's examine a situation that occurs frequently on the unit and consider possible aggressive, assertive, and nonassertive responses with regard to their possible costs and benefits.

You are working the day shift, and a fellow staff member approaches you at the medication cart while you're pouring 12:00 meds. The staff member has to move a patient at the other end of the hall and says, "I'd like you to help me move Mr. M. into a new room so that we can get an admission."

Identify the costs and benefits for each of the possible responses given below:

Aggressive:
"That's crazy! I am doing meds, and you'll have to find someone else."

Costs of Aggressive Response:

_____

_____

Benefits of Aggressive Response:

_____

_____

Assertive:
"I need to pour these meds, but I will help in 10 minutes if you can wait."

Costs of Assertive Response:

_____

_____

Benefits of Assertive Response:

_____

_____

Nonassertive:
"Well, . . . I can help if it won't take long."

Costs of Nonassertive Response:

_____

_____

Benefits of Nonassertive Response:

_____

_____

One way to be more in control of your responses is to use the Inner Action Model (chapter 1) to determine whether your actions or statements will be aggressive, assertive, or nonassertive. Using the example above, let's imagine what you might have been thinking and feeling before each of those responses.

Example

"I'd like you to help me move Mr. M. . . ."

Thought: That's outrageous! I would never ask that!
Feelings: Self-righteousness.
Action: Aggression.

Thought: I have the right to finish the meds. She needs help, too.
Feelings: Being in control, making a rational response.
Action: Assertive.

Thought: I'd better do it, or she won't like me.
Feelings: Resentfulness, inadequacy.
Action: Nonassertive.

Obviously, one way to change your behavior and become more assertive is to tune in to your thoughts and feelings. If you are thinking and feeling in ways that lead to the Self-Defeating Zone, you are unlikely to behave in assertive ways. Limited self-awareness throws people into aggressive or passive behavior, because they are unaware of the intensity of their feelings, or because they're confused about their own intentions. Self-awareness also minimizes the possibilities of misinterpretation that can lead to conflict.

Inventory

The inventory shown in figure 4-2 is included to help you understand more fully the ways in which you interact and communicate. Once you complete the inventory, use the Inventory Process Sheet (figure 4-3) to look for patterns in your ways of relating and for situations where you respond with aggressive, assertive, or nonassertive behaviors. You will be able to use your answers to these questions when you begin to work with the actual skills of assertive behavior.

Figure 4-2. Assertiveness Inventory

	How Assertive Are You? Please circle the number that best fits your response.				
	I'm Not at All Likely to Do This			I'm Very Likely to Do This	
1. Your boss has asked you to do more work than you can realistically accomplish. Instead of taking on this burden, you share your feelings with her/him.	1	2	3	4	5
2. You see one of your coworkers slipping up on a job and you confront this person about their behavior.	1	2	3	4	5
3. You let a coworker know that you feel he/she is using your friendship by pressuring you to do some of her/his work.	1	2	3	4	5
4. You let someone close to you know that you feel you're doing more work in the relationship than they are.	1	2	3	4	5
5. You say no to social invitations that you're not interested in accepting.	1	2	3	4	5
6. You resist sales pressure.	1	2	3	4	5
7. You send back food in a restaurant when it's unacceptable.	1	2	3	4	5
8. You feel you're due for a raise and you ask for it.	1	2	3	4	5
9. You need help to complete your work on a project and you ask your boss to help you.	1	2	3	4	5
10. You're working on a committee and you feel strongly that many members are leading the group in a direction that is wrong. You let them know how you feel.	1	2	3	4	5
11. There is a coworker whose lack of tact is getting the group into difficulty. You confront him/her directly instead of dealing with it behind their back.	1	2	3	4	5
12. You let your boss know you've been wrongly accused of a slip-up.	1	2	3	4	5
13. You let an individual know that you have seen them steal hospital property.	1	2	3	4	5
14. You compliment a coworker on a job well done.	1	2	3	4	5

Continued on next page

Figure 4-2. (Continued)

	How Assertive Are You? Please circle the number that best fits your response.				
	I'm Not at All Likely to Do This				I'm Very Likely to Do This
15. You initiate an apology when you think you're at fault.	1	2	3	4	5
16. When you're working in a new area or with new material, you ask for feedback from those you work with.	1	2	3	4	5
17. You let someone know that what they forgot to do for you was important.	1	2	3	4	5
18. You let someone who is always late know how you feel about this.	1	2	3	4	5
19. Someone at work is making sexual advances toward you. You let them know that you don't appreciate this and want to be treated in a more professional and less "familiar" manner.	1	2	3	4	5
20. When someone's behavior indicates that you might have offended them, you check this out to see if you read them right.	1	2	3	4	5
21. You request the prompt return of borrowed items or loaned money.	1	2	3	4	5
22. You continue to converse with someone who disagrees with you.	1	2	3	4	5
23. When you become aware of something that might help a coworker or a patient, you speak up and follow through, even if others ignore it because they think it's a hassle or not their job.	1	2	3	4	5

Source: Reprinted, with permission, from "Tactful Assertiveness" Workshop Materials, The Einstein Consulting Group, 1982.

Figure 4-3. Inventory Process Sheet

Directions: Answer these questions using your responses on the Assertiveness Inventory.

1. In what situations or with which people do you feel comfortable being assertive?
2. In what situations or with which people do you find it difficult to be assertive?
3. What do you think causes your nonassertive behavior?
4. Describe a situation in which you would like to be more assertive.

You will be able to use your answers to these questions when you begin to work with the actual skills of assertive behavior.

The Risks

Change is always accompanied by risk. What risks might you encounter by becoming more assertive?

Some of the risks associated with becoming assertive include the following:

1. **You might not choose the perfect response.** Despite what etiquette books tell us, there is no perfect social response to any one situation. You want to find a response that works—that's good enough. As a beginner, you also have to allow for mistakes or failures. Keep practicing!
2. **You might not get what you want, even if you are assertive.** There is no guarantee of success. Being assertive simply improves the chances that you will get what you want and that you will feel good about yourself.
3. **Some people won't like your new behavior.** If you've been nonassertive in your relationships in the past, some of your friends and coworkers will be surprised by your new assertiveness, and some may not like it. Some of their negative reactions might be due to unexpected change. You will have to decide whether feeling good about yourself and getting what you want are worth that risk. You can acknowledge the change in your own behavior without becoming defensive (and aggressive) or nonassertive. In time, friends and coworkers may come to respect you more.

It takes time to change. If you try being assertive only once or twice and then evaluate on that basis whether you really want to be assertive, you'll probably decide it was a mistake. Plan to allow at least several attempts at being assertive! After all, how long did it take you to learn to be nonassertive?

Your Rights and Responsibilities

Knowing your rights will support your assertive behavior. In *The Assertive Option: Your Rights and Responsibilities* (Research Press, 1978, pp. 80–81), Patricia Jakubowski and Arthur J. Lange listed 10 basic rights that you—and all people—have. The following list is adapted from their materials:

1. **The right to act in ways that promote your dignity and self-respect.** Each of us is given the right to decide our values and life-style as long as we don't violate the rights of others. You have the right to be yourself and to act in ways

that promote your self-respect. When you feel good about yourself and accept this basic right, you will enjoy your relationships more. And you'll be able to deal more easily with others whose actions impinge on your rights—in ways that acknowledge their rights as well.

2. **The right to be treated with respect.** You have the right to be treated with respect by every person with whom you interact. Mutual respect promotes equality in relationships and allows each person the opportunity to feel good and to grow.

3. **The right to experience and express your thoughts and feelings.** Human beings are emotive creatures. Emotions are responsible for much of the depth and richness in our lives. Emotions are neither good nor bad; they simply exist. Instead of accepting that, your self-talk may include statements such as, "I shouldn't feel angry, sad, lonely, or anxious," or, "It's wrong to feel jealous," or, "I shouldn't be so shy." You have every right to experience your feelings. You also have a right to express your feelings in ways that respect the rights of others. Censoring your emotions and responsible expression often leads to nonassertive behavior, self-deprecation, and feelings of inadequacy. It's important that you care for yourself in ways that are responsible and that keep you out of the Self-Defeating Zone.

4. **The right to slow down and make conscious decisions before you act.** You have the right to tune into your thoughts and feelings before you act. Sometimes this requires a moment, and sometimes it means postponing a decision for some time. You will not take care of yourself responsibly if you respond spontaneously with automatic answers and decisions. Take the time you need.

5. **The right to ask for what you want.** If you are respectful of the rights of others, what could you want from them that you can't feel free to ask for? You can ask for anything; of course, that doesn't automatically mean that you will get it. "But," you say, "I feel guilty asking for what I want." We've already established that you are responsible for yourself; other people are responsible for themselves, too. Let them answer you responsibly for themselves. "But," you say, "I might be rejected, refused, or hurt." Sure, you may not get what you ask for; that's the risk you take. But you'll never get what you don't ask for.

6. **The right to say no.** If you do not want to do something, you have the right to say no. This right is inherent. Saying

no does not make you a bad person. The other person's right to ask you for what they want is no greater than your right to say no—or yes, for that matter. You and others have the right to ask for what you want and to answer honestly when asked. Sometimes, people will not like your answer, but that doesn't mean that they don't like you personally, that they will never ask you for anything else again, or that they'll retaliate against you.

7. **The right to change your mind.** You have the right to change your mind after you have given additional thought to a matter. Many contracts allow a grace period for you to rethink a decision that is legally binding. It's important that you exercise this right when you want to change your mind.

8. **The right not to be perfect.** Everyone wants to do the best they can at whatever they undertake. But not everyone can be perfect at *everything* they have to do. You have the right to do the best you're capable of, even if it isn't 100 percent on every task all the time. Sometimes, trying to be the best at everything means doing for others at the expense of doing for yourself.

9. **The right to make mistakes.** You need to give yourself an allowance for error. It's not the end of the world if you make a mistake. Mistakes are inevitable. Although you can do many things to avoid mistakes, you may still make them. Beating yourself up will probably do nothing to help you avoid making future mistakes. And it will surely land you in the Self-Defeating Zone. If you are going to try being more assertive, you will make some mistakes, and you need to allow for them as a natural part of learning and growth.

10. **The right to feel good about yourself.** Many people find it difficult to say positive things about themselves, to accept compliments, and to report their successes. You don't have to think of it as bragging. Talking honestly about your accomplishments is fine. Likewise, there's nothing to be gained by going out of your way to emphasize your weaknesses to others. You have the right to experience your self-worth and to express it to others.

Here are some other rights you have that you might want to consider exercising more often (*The Assertive Option: Your Rights and Responsibilities*, pp. 80–81):

- I have a right to be treated as an individual with my own special values, skills, and needs.
- I have the right to have this uniqueness respected.

- I have the right to my own feelings and opinions.
- I have the right to say "I don't know."
- I have the right to feel angry.
- I have the right to make decisions regarding my own life.
- I have the right to recognize that my needs are as important as the needs of others.

These rights are the foundation of assertive behavior. To become more assertive, you will want to become very familiar with these rights. Put copies of them in places where you can review them daily. For example, you might put a copy on your mirror and take a minute in the morning to review each one. Try saying the rights out loud—and say them with confidence.

Once you know the 10 rights and have adopted them as *your rights,* begin by focusing on 1 or 2 with which you feel comfortable. As you go through the day, you will encounter situations to which these rights apply and in which you would like to be more assertive. Tune in to what you say to yourself about each right. In what ways do you stop yourself from asserting your rights? Now, try to balance any disabling statements or feelings with this sentence: "I may (think, feel) and I . . . (complete the statement with your right)."

For example, if you say to yourself, "I really should say yes to this request instead of no," when you do not want to comply, you might balance that thought with, "I may think I should say yes; however, I have a right to say no."

As you read and recite each of these rights, practice listening or tuning in your thoughts and feelings, and use the balancing statement to correct old disabling messages you've learned. Use the exercises on the preceding pages to see clearly how your previous thoughts and feelings have caused your behavior to be nonassertive or aggressive. You can also use the list given in figure 4-4 to help you tune in to your old thoughts and to develop new ways of thinking more assertively.

Figure 4-4. Assessing the Assertive Situation

1. Describe a situation in which you'd like to be more assertive.
2. What do you want from that situation? What would you like to be different? What would you like to change?
3. What keeps you from doing something about the situation? (What are the self-statements, thoughts, emotions, irrational beliefs?)
4. Develop alternatives to those thoughts—ask yourself: "Are they 100 percent true?" "How terrible would a negative consequence be?"

Source: Reprinted, with permission, from "Tactful Assertiveness" Workshop Materials, The Einstein Consulting Group, 1982.

Now you can begin to act on your rights. Start with the rights you are comfortable with and practice with smaller issues. Use the statements that are discussed in the next section of this chapter. As you become more comfortable with these assertive behaviors and actions, move to the rights you feel less secure about. In this way, you can recall your successes with new assertive behaviors you have already used.

Seven Basic Assertive Messages

Most messages we send to people about their behavior are "you" messages—messages directed to other people that are likely to make them feel uncomfortable and resistant to change. Some examples of "you" messages include "Stop doing that," "Leave her alone," "You are acting like a juvenile," or "You are driving me crazy." "You" messages also take the form of threats: "You'd better . . . or I'll . . . ."

An "I" message, on the other hand, allows a person who is affected by the behavior of another to express the impact it has on her or him. At the same time, it leaves the responsibility for modifying the behavior with the person who demonstrated it. By making an assertive statement, you cut to the core of an issue and handle differences without blaming, demanding, or defending.

You can use seven basic assertive "I" messages as a guide to changing your present communication and behavior. For each message, we have identified its purpose, some examples, and likely results and tips:

1. **"I want" statement.**
   Purpose: This type of statement helps clarify what you want both to yourself and to others. It tells others what you want to do or what you want them to do. Where their needs conflict with yours, negotiation to achieve a compromise can be done more easily.
   Examples:
   - "I want to know what I did to make you angry, but I don't want you to call me names."
   - "I'd like you to be on time when you have a meeting with me."
   - "I'd like you to help me with a dressing change sometime before 10:00 a.m. Is that possible?"
   - "I'd really appreciate it if you would talk with Mrs. S; she is very concerned about her husband's condition. Could you do that today?"

Results: Others know *how* to fulfill your wants. Even if the person doesn't want to respond, you've expressed your want. Now problem solving or negotiation can take place.

Tips:

- Tell the person how intensely you want this. Perhaps quantify the importance. (For example, "I want you to stop pressuring me about trying for that promotion; that's a 10 on a scale from 1 to 10!")
- State what your request means and what it doesn't mean. (For example, "I'd like you to finish this week. If you can't, it will be inconvenient, although not disastrous.")
- Be as exact as possible in stating what you want. If you need to state a limitation you have, don't criticize yourself. (For example, "I need help to figure out this dosage" rather than "I always screw up these calculations.")
- Avoid negative talk and unnecessary flattery. Be prepared to offer a compromise or to negotiate a trade-off.

2. **"I feel" statement.**

Purpose: "I feel" statements help you to express your feelings without causing the other person to feel inadequate or inferior. When you state clearly what you feel, you may help to reduce misunderstandings about your feelings. It's very easy to misinterpret behavioral or nonverbal messages about feelings. Verbal statements provide helpful information to others, and they can use this information to make a response.

Examples:

- "I feel grateful for your help with this patient."
- "I feel much safer knowing there will be two of us on the unit tonight."
- "I feel overwhelmed when you spend the first 10 minutes of your report complaining about how difficult the patient care was the night before."

Results: These statements help you to express your feelings without attacking the self-esteem of the other person. You give the other person important information that he or she may want to act on.

Tips: Be as specific as you can. Use words that describe the degree of your feelings so that you will be accurate and clearly understood.

3. **"Mixed feelings" statement.**

Purpose: Sometimes you have both positive and negative—opposite—feelings about an issue, event, or situation. Rather than remaining silent or presenting only one feeling, it's useful to state both. In stating both feelings, it's helpful to tell where both feelings are coming from. This will help to further clarify your message.

Examples:

- "I'm happy to get a salary increase, and I appreciate that you've noticed my work. But I feel disappointed and annoyed that my raise still puts my salary below that of men here in the same position."
- "I am grateful that you granted my request for time off at Christmas rather than at New Year's this year. But I feel frustrated about having only one day off, because I can't go out of town to visit my parents. If we work together on the schedule, is there any way I could have my two days off in conjunction with the holiday?"

Results: You have a chance of being understood and influencing the other person. People with mixed feelings too often say nothing.

Tips: You might choose to share one feeling and get feedback on it before introducing the second. Just make sure that you express both.

4. **"Flat-out no" statement.**

   Purpose: The "flat-out no" statement will state clearly and emphatically that the answer is no.

   Examples:

   - "No."
   - "As I said, the answer is no!"

   Results: You will not comply with the request.

   Tips: Before you say no, be sure that is what you want to say. If you are unsure, indicate that you'll need time to think about it. If you need more information, ask questions in order to get the complete picture before answering. Keep your answer short, and remember that reasons and excuses give the other person something to argue about. You don't owe the person an explanation. In fact, you may not even be sure why you want to say no—and that is your right. If the person argues with you, repeat your answer and shake your head to say no at the same time.

5. **Empathetic assertion.**

   Purpose: This type of statement is used when you want to convey sensitivity to or understanding of the other person's situation and, at the same time, to state what you are feeling. Conveying recognition does not imply agreement or sympathy. It simply indicates that you acknowledge an awareness of the other person's circumstances. The statement also gives you the opportunity to clarify your feelings.

Examples:
- "Doctor, I know it's hard for you to say when you'll be making rounds, but I would like to be available to discuss some of my concerns about the patient's recovery."
- "I can see that you are frustrated because you didn't get the tray you ordered for dinner. At the moment I can't solve that problem, but I will call dietary for you right now."
- "I know what the cost of a room is here per day, but answering such requests is not part of our duties as nurses."

Results: Other people know where you stand. They also feel understood. This reduces the likelihood of defensiveness or hostility on their parts.

Tips:
- Keep your empathy statement brief. Otherwise, you and the other person lose sight of your feelings and wants.
- Avoid gimmicky, empty phrases such as "I know how you feel."
- Be specific about what you understand. (For example, "I realize you feel hurt by my criticism.")

6. **Confrontational assertion.**

Purpose: When someone says that they will do something, but fails to, this type of assertion helps you to clarify what was said and what you want now or in the future.

Examples:
- "When I applied for this position, you stated that I would not have more than three patients per shift. The supervisor consistently expects me to carry a heavier patient load, and I want you to clarify your agreement with her today."
- "You said that you wanted to hear our feelings about how the unit is managed, but you never act on any of our suggestions. I'd like to bring this up for discussion at the next staff meeting."

Results: When you are descriptive about the person's behavior, instead of being judgmental, the person is less likely to act defensive. You aren't attacking the person—you're describing the behavior.

Tips: Point out the discrepancy instead of angrily confronting the person. Find out what happened and why. Avoid jumping to conclusions.

7. **"I" message statement.**

Purpose: This message is especially useful for expressing difficult negative feelings, giving the person feedback on how their actions affected you. Stating a specific concrete effect that person's behavior had on you will make the impact of the message more effective and positive.

Format:
When you . . . .
I feel . . . .
Because . . . .
I want . . . .

Examples:
* "Dr. Smith, when you start yelling in the nurses' station like this, I feel humiliated and angry. I am willing to listen to what you are concerned about, but I want you to stop yelling at me."
* "Mary, when you become insistent that I work a double shift by asking me repeatedly to change my plans, I feel pressured and resentful. I know you feel pressed to have enough staff, but I want you to stop asking me three or four times to work extra. If I can work, I will tell you the first time."

Results: People clearly see the results or consequences of their specific behavior. They can decide whether or not to change.

Tips: It helps to plan ahead—thinking through and even writing down a solid "I" message.

As you begin to work with each of these messages, use the Guide to Assertive Planning (figure 4-5). This will help you to plan for situations in which you want to be more assertive and will increase the likelihood of your success.

As you practice using assertive messages, remember to demonstrate assertive body language. Here are some points to consider:

* Maintain direct eye contact.
* Keep your body posture erect.

Figure 4-5. Guide to Assertive Planning

1. Specify the situation
2. Set goals and subgoals.
3. Identify your personal rights.
4. Change irrational thinking to rational, supportive thinking.
5. Plan assertive language.
6. Carry out the plan.
7. Assess how you did and decide what's next.

Source: Reprinted, with permission, from "Tactful Assertiveness" Workshop Materials, The Einstein Consulting Group, 1982.

- Speak clearly and audibly.
- Don't plead.
- Use gestures and facial expressions for emphasis.
- Use appropriate timing.

What If They Don't Agree?

Just because you're assertive doesn't mean you will always get what you want the first time you try—you may not even get it at all. The other person has the same rights you have and may have other needs. That does not mean you have to back down. Sometimes you will need to compromise and negotiate an acceptable outcome. However, there will also be times when you do not want to compromise. Here are some interactive skills that will help you in those circumstances.

The Broken Record

This technique requires simple persistence and repetition of your "I" message without getting irritated, angry, or loud. Here are some tips:

- Don't get bogged down in excessive words.
- Don't give up.
- Don't be swayed by anything the person says.
- Repeat yourself in a calm voice.

Figure 4-6 demonstrates the use of the broken record technique to get what you want.

Fogging

This technique requires you to agree with the statements of the other person as much as possible, until the other person gives up and goes away. For example:
"You look terrible today."
"I guess I do."
"Look at your hair! When did you have it curled last?"
"Yeah, it could use a perm."
"You'll never get ahead in life looking like that."
"You're probably right."
This technique is especially useful when you've tried everything else and failed.

Figure 4-6. Example of the Broken Record Technique

Sharon visited a major department store and bought two blouses and three pairs of shoes. When she got home and unpacked her bags, she found that one gray shoe was streaked along the side. Sharon, receipt and gray shoes in hand, returned to the department store and confronted the clerk:

Sharon: When I was here earlier, I bought these shoes. When I got home, I found that one of them is streaked along the side. I'm bringing them back to return them. I want my money back.

Clerk: I'm sorry, but our policy does not allow returns. I can give you credit toward another pair of shoes.

Sharon: You don't seem to understand. These shoes are damaged. I want my money back.

Clerk: We can't give you your money back, but we can give you another pair of shoes at the same price. Would you like to see other shoes?

Sharon: I don't want another pair of shoes. I want to return these, and I want my money back.

Clerk: Well, I'm not authorized to return your money.

Sharon: Then, can I see the manager?

The clerk summoned the manager. Sharon showed him the damaged shoes.

Manager: I understand what the problem is, but I'm sorry, our policy only allows for exchanges or credit.

Sharon: But I don't want an exchange or a credit. I want my money back.

Manager: I'm sorry, but . . . .

Sharon: I'm sorry, too. These shoes were damaged before I left the store. This is the pair I wanted, and I won't accept a substitute. I want my money back.

Manager: Well, perhaps we can make this exception. (He turns to the clerk.) Give this woman her money back.

Unhooking

When you use an "I" message, the other person may respond with reasons why they cannot do what you are asking. The technique in unhooking is not to get caught up in their reasons. You need to express your "I" message again and again until you are unwilling to discuss it further.

For example, you may have been asked to do something that you are unskilled in, that is not part of your job, or that violates an existing policy or procedure. Although the other person may have several reasons why you should do what they want despite your objections, you need to stay "unhooked" and repeat your statement:

Doctor: "Please give this med I.V. every 3 hours."

Nurse: "We are not permitted to administer the medication I.V."

Doctor: "They do it for me on the other floors. I don't like your refusal to carry out my order."

Nurse: "I cannot account for what happens on other floors. On this floor, I am not permitted to give the drug I.V. Perhaps you would like to talk to my nurse manager."

Here's another example. A nurse working the evening shift is approached by the supervisor to work a double shift.

Nurse: "Hi, Jane."

Supervisor: "Hi. I need to talk with you about nights. They are short two people. Can you work?"

Nurse: "No, Jane."

Supervisor: "I know you've been busy, but you'll leave them in an unsafe situation if you don't work. I can't get anyone to come in."

Nurse: "I'm sorry, Jane, but I simply can't work tonight."

Supervisor: "If it's a scheduling problem, I'll work on it."

Nurse: "No, I have a commitment for tonight, and I can't work."

Supervisor: "But surely you don't want the unit to be that short."

Nurse: "No, I don't want that. I can see that you are trying very hard to fill the hole, but I just can't work tonight."

Summary

This chapter has attempted to provide you with the basic knowledge and beginning skills to communicate clearly and assertively with others on the job about your thoughts, feelings, and wants. The importance of stepping into your personal power through assertive behavior is truly the message of this chapter. You've seen how many of the feelings of frustration, anger, and powerlessness can be positively managed if you have the skill to know what to say and how to say it. This chapter not only reminds you that you are in the driver's seat, but also gives you the instructions on how to operate the control board—the *assertive* control board.

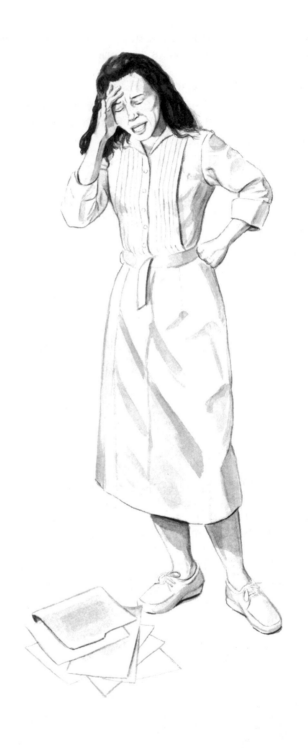

Chapter 5

Stress: A Critical Course

The following scenario may sound familiar: You roll over and hit the alarm, deciding "just 5 more minutes." Five minutes turns into 20 minutes. You start your whole day rushed! You throw on your uniform and discover that one sleeve is a mass of wrinkles. You burn the toast. As you fly out the door, you remember that you forgot your watch. At this point, your insides feel like scrambled eggs!

Once you're in the car, you flip on the radio . . . just in time for a news brief. Another military crisis is heating up, the stock market is down, a large plane crashes, and, locally, a child is missing. But, that's not all—the main expressway has a construction detour. That does it!

You arrive at work, and as you walk onto the floor, you're greeted with, "Guess what! We're short-staffed again!" Everyone is running around the unit like an evacuation team. After hearing the report— Mr. Smith had a bad night, three pre-ops need to be done, and the obese patient in Room 301, who needs an army to move him, has to be moved again—you're exhausted before you begin. You thought you could handle two courses instead of one this semester. You think, "If I get through this morning, let alone class tonight, it will be a miracle."

Feeling overwhelmed, frustrated, out of control, and ready to explode from the pressure? It's called *stress*.

A low level of stress is healthy; it's a stimulant and a motivator. It's the stuff that challenges us. But on too many days and in too many ways, the stress you're under as a nurse seems downright absurd. It's time to put on the brakes. It's time to find your own inner harmony in the midst of this crazy, stressful world of nursing.

What Is Stress?

What does the word *stress* bring to mind? Tension, annoyance, fearful situations, feeling uncertain and inadequate, unrealistic work loads, accidents, demands, responsibilities, deadlines, and expectations. These are responses that nurses gave when we asked them to define stress. What would you add to the list?

Most people respond to stress negatively. They focus on its undesirable aspects, or "distress." Dr. Hans Selye of Montreal, the world's foremost stress researcher, defines stress as a "nonspecific response of the body to any demand made on it." Selye regards stress as a neutral physiological phenomenon, devoid of "good" or "bad" value. It's the meaning we assign to the external event that determines whether this physiological reaction is an energy boost or an energy drain.

The first fact to digest about stress is that it is a *neutral, natural, and normal* response of the body to any external situation that places a demand on the body's energy resources. That includes most life situations. Pleasure, joy, happiness, and excitement also trigger the body's stress response, but because we do not see these as undesirable and do not seek to avoid them, the energy drain is less, and we do not experience these emotions as "stressful."

So, if you see stress as negative, it's time to expand your view. Let's look at the "stress" model, according to Professional Renewal:

Trigger events ⟶ Response ⟶ Stress
(External situations)   (Assigned meaning)   (Outcome or result)

On the left are the events that trigger stress—that is, the new baby, the flat tire, the fuel bill, short-staffing, and working a double shift. On the far right is the outcome or result of the way we process the event; that is, feeling upset or anxious, crying, or experiencing your heart pounding, a knot in your stomach, or a headache. Between the trigger events and the stress outcome is the **response.** *Herein lies the key to managing stress.* Stress falls between the ears or in the mind. Stress is often referred to as an "inside" job. Here's why: Your internal response to an event is what results in stress, not the event itself. It's the meaning you assign to the trigger event that determines whether you'll feel happy, sad, anxious, trapped, or free.

Consider the following example. See how the same event can trigger two very different responses. One is "eustress," a positive response to stress, and the other "distress," a negative response:

- **Nurse A is given a promotion.** To this nurse, it's terrific news; she feels challenged, stimulated, and motivated to take on new responsibilities. She's excited about discovering a whole new side of herself.

- **Nurse B is also given a promotion.** He, on the other hand, is ambivalent about the news of a job promotion. This nurse feels worried, insecure, and inadequate, wondering "Will I be able to do it?" Nurse B is not looking forward to making the necessary adjustments.

The same event has triggered two opposite responses.

Now, proceed to the next step. What would you expect Nurse A to feel? Excitement, new energy, eagerness to move ahead. How about Nurse B? Confusion, low energy, an inclination to limp along. So, the event—a job promotion—is neutral until the mind assigns a meaning to it. That meaning depends on how you choose to record or interpret the event. *It's your choice!*

Once again you see the word *choice.* Most of us are so used to having an automatic response to circumstances or events that we short-circuit the internal thought process that lies between the event and our response—which is where the choice really lies.

The key: *Choosing* your thoughts and *choosing* your feelings in response to life events. No one else but you can control your stress.

Are you thinking, "Yes, *but* . . . look at the conditions we work under in nursing"? It is true that working conditions are difficult and demanding. However, the way you internalize the external is what produces stressful feelings of frustration, guilt, helplessness, anger, and exhaustion. It might help you to think about how your coworkers respond to stress. Who, in your opinion, handles stress exceptionally well? Who, on the other hand, falls apart or comes unglued? Here you have two nurses, with the same work conditions, and yet totally different responses. Does this mean that the nurse who handles stress exceptionally well is thrilled about the staffing shortage? Does it mean that she doesn't care as much as the nurse who comes unglued? No! What it means is that she knows how to use energy. She knows how not to drag herself down with negative, destructive responses to stress. She exercises wise choices.

Consider another example. You're stuck in traffic. Do you get angry, curse the other drivers, bark at your passengers, bang your fist on the steering wheel, and work yourself into a throbbing headache? Do you justify your behavior by blaming that idiot up ahead for a car breakdown? Or, do your rationalize your behavior by saying, "I hate traffic. I can't control my anger. This always drives me crazy."

Stop and ask yourself, "Is my response appropriate? Dysfunctional? Life-enhancing? Physically and emotionally disabling? Do

I have any control over the traffic jam? Is it an intelligent decision to use my life-energy festering about something over which I have absolutely no control?" Probably not!

So why not decide to *respond differently?* What if you choose to use your mind and energy in *enabling* instead of disabling ways? You can reprogram your response with a flip of a switch. It's a matter of making a *decision* to do so. Try new behaviors in a traffic jam. Listen to a new radio station. Construct in your mind the letter you need to write. Sing, whistle, or plan your dinner menu for the week. Or simply take a deep breath, relax, and go with the flow.

You don't have to like traffic, but you can learn to suspend your anger and conserve your energy by recognizing that you have no control over the situation. Also, you can nip in the bud the physical tension, headache, and general wear and tear on your body that result from a full-blown negative response.

The Professional Renewal Concept: Change the things you can change and let go of things you can't.

The Power of Awareness

The first step in managing stress is *awareness.* Being aware of your emotional and physical self helps you take charge of your reactions. Each of us has a choice to respond to the needs we have emotionally and physically, or to ignore those needs.

Consider this powerful thought contained in *The Three Pillars of Zen* (New York, Anchor Books, 1980, pp. 10–11). Philip Kapleau recounts the following story about Zen Master Ikkyu:

One day a man of the people said to Zen Master Ikkyu, "Master, will you please write for me some maxims of the highest wisdom?" Ikkyu immediately took his brush and wrote the word "Attention."

"Is that all?" asked the man. "Will you not add something more?"

Ikkyu then wrote twice running, "Attention. Attention."

"Well," remarked the man rather irritably, "I really don't see much depth or subtlety in what you have just written."

Then Ikkyu wrote the same word three times running, "Attention. Attention. Attention."

Half-angered, the man demanded, "What does that word 'Attention' mean anyway?"

And Ikkyu answered gently, "Attention means attention."

Paying attention may seem like a very simple thing when you examine the stress epidemic among nurses. When you pay attention to stress, you begin to notice the choices you have, and you realize the extent of your own power and control. Working without tension is a choice—it's an attitude to commit yourself to. Pay attention to the choices you make about stress, and exercise the control you have over your health, well-being, and happiness.

Our Physical Response to Stress

Now let's look more closely at your body's physiological response to stress. Bodily reaction to stress affects all the major systems of your body, including your autonomic nervous and endocrine systems. Simply put, these systems combine to speed up the cardiovascular functions, creating adrenaline secretions that cause a rush of energy to the muscles and heart and, at the same time, slow down the gastrointestinal function. This process interrupts the digestive process because your entire body has turned its resources in the direction of the perceived threat. Turning on your stress alarm frequently and over long periods of time causes wear and tear on your body and increases the likelihood of illness, contributing to slow degenerative diseases that surface over time.

The perception of a threat is often what sends stress into motion. Our ancestors encountered many more physical threats than we experience, such as wild animals that physically threatened their safety. Today, most threats are unrelated to life-or-death situations. Although we face fewer wild animals, our minds and egos struggle for control over our environment. Instead of lions, tigers, and bears, our systems are assaulted by discourtesies, insults, disappointments, and annoyances—sometimes real, sometimes perceived. Recent research reveals that, although we might perceive a threat, we often hold ourselves in check, not releasing the physical energy behind our negative response to a perceived threat. This repressed or unexpressed energy triggers physical tension that backs up and negatively taxes our bodies.

Here's an analogy to help you visualize what actually happens. Imagine a firehouse when the alarm goes off. Remember how it was done in the old movies? The fire fighters jump out of bed and into their clothes, slide down the fire pole, leap into the fire truck, and speed away to extinguish the fire. Once they get to the fire, they slam on the brakes, jump off the truck, pull out the long, winding hose, and stack up the tall ladders. Then, all of a sudden someone yells, "Stop . . . it's a false alarm!" Even though no fire occurred, didn't the fire fighters experience the same degree of both physical wear and tear (running, rushing, jumping, and speeding) and emotional wear and tear (fear of being burned or killed in the fire) that they would have experienced if there had been a fire? Of course!

And so do you, every time your "stress alarms" go off. You send out the fire engines and gear up your biological systems every time you perceive a threat. And most of the time, the "threat" that precipitates this response is not physical but psychological. Your body often experiences false alarms of this sort.

Consider these two scenarios:

Scene 1: The doctor glares at you. The doctor's words begin to pour out in angry tones. "You must have gone to school? I gather they taught you to read English. This order is written in English . . . see . . . and I suggest you get this medication up here now and into this patient STAT before she dies!"

Scene 2: You feel like a balloon blown up to full capacity, and you're ready to burst. You storm out of the patient's room blurting, "Why is this patient yelling at me? I'm only trying to help him! All he does is complain. I know his situation is difficult, but I don't even want to go in there anymore. I've had it!"

Sound familiar? Count yourself among the lucky few if you don't recognize these scenarios. According to Gloria Farraro Donnelly, R.N., M.S.W., chairman of the department of nursing at LaSalle University in Philadelphia, study after study has shown that one of the most frequent causes of stress in any nurse's work environment is just this kind of breakdown in interpersonal relations.

Reconsider the two scenes above. How do you know when it's appropriate to pull your stress alarm and call out the fire engines? Ask yourself the following questions to get a handle on whether your response is a rational and appropriate one:

1. Is your life physically in danger?   ☐ Yes   ☐ No

2. Based on your prior experience, is   ☐ Yes   ☐ No
   it likely this storm will subside?

3. Will your performance or ability to   ☐ Yes   ☐ No
   respond to these situations be further
   enhanced by gearing your body up for
   a stress response?

4. Are you willing to pay the price of   ☐ Yes   ☐ No
   having stress cause you physical
   damage or emotional disturbance?

The next time you find yourself in the midst of a potentially stressful situation, check yourself. Decide whether you really want to pull your stress alarm. After asking yourself the preceding questions, you may decide to pass instead of pull.

Stress Signals

The first step in managing stress is to recognize stress in yourself. Many nurses become so accustomed to stress that the absence of tension may well feel foreign. True relaxation is a rare commodity. Nurses who go home after work with a splitting headache or sleep the evening away probably aren't attuned to early signs and symptoms that would have allowed them to ward off debilitating stress attacks.

Stress signals range from the very subtle to dramatic and life-threatening bodily breakdowns. There are four stages in the progression:

Stage 1: Tap-Tap
Stage 2: Knock-Knock
Stage 3: Bang-Bang
Stage 4: Clobber-Clobber

Stage 1: Tap-Tap

This is like a gentle tap on the shoulder. During the first stage, the state of your mind is exceedingly important. If it's calm and clear, you can hear the faint voice of tension and anxiety in time to do something about it. Possible examples: choosing to eat lightly at lunch so that you can avoid sluggishness during afternoon work or catching yourself before you get caught in the trap of trading "ain't it awful" stories with your coworkers or replacing your tight shoes—even though you love their looks—with your old, comfortable standbys so that you won't be limping by the end of your shift.

These are examples of tuning in to your instinctive capacity for self-guidance. Once again, you have a choice. You can respond to stress signals, you can postpone your response, or you can ignore these signals indefinitely. The first course of action is preventive and will nip stress in the bud.

Stage 2: Knock-Knock

This stage is an obvious knock at your door. Sporadic pain begins to appear. If you've chosen to ignore the subtle signs of the Tap-Tap stage, the inner signals of pain, discomfort, distress, and tension intensify. For example, if you ignore your first sign of a need to urinate, pressure on the bladder increases to the point where you must pay attention and respond to it. Another example: If you've been allowing frustration and irritation to move in on you inch by inch all day long, and you've postponed responding to early signs of tension, then your body will escalate its signal of the need to release tension by a headache, backache, or upset stomach. This is your body's way of getting your attention—"knock-knock"—to let you know that your body is out of balance and needs you to restore it to equilibrium.

These tension indicators can be clearly physical, like occasional mild pain, indigestion, colds, elevated blood pressure, rapid heartbeat; or mental, like irritability, forgetfulness, inability to concentrate, and abruptness with patients and coworkers.

At this stage, many people fall into the trap of treating the symptoms and overlooking the root cause. You reach for antacid, aspirin, and tranquilizers, and camouflage the pain while you continue to put excessive strain on your physical and emotional self. Thus, the "state of imbalance" is further aggravated. So far, you've succeeded in ignoring the signals of both Tap-Tap and Knock-Knock.

The Concept: The earlier you respond to a physical or emotional need, the less effort it takes to rectify the imbalance, and the greater the results. Remember, an ounce of prevention is worth a pound of cure.

Stage 3: Bang-Bang

Imagine a sledgehammer whacking at your door. In this Bang-Bang stage, alarming and disturbing long-term pain and disability command attention. If you failed to heed the warnings in the two earlier stages, this is the point when your body aggressively communicates to you the damage you are causing to your physical and emotional health. More serious and persistent pain and illness begin to manifest themselves, crying out for your urgent attention.

The occasional headache has now turned into the chronic migraine. The minor stomach upset has turned into the first signs of a peptic ulcer. Bouts of high blood pressure, now more regular, have developed into symptoms of cardiac disease. Tightness and stiffness have turned into early stages of arthritis. Before you know it, *you* need the hospital bed.

You've been out of touch with your body. Chances are, you're experiencing a rude awakening. You can't keep pushing, pushing, pushing and not expect something to snap, break, or wear out!

You're not feeling well, and this depletes your energy. Your diminished energy affects your job performance, and you become more tense and afraid. This creates a vicious circle that further drains your physical, emotional, and even financial resources.

Stage 4: Clobber-Clobber

At this stage, you're being hit in the back of the head by a two-by-four. You've ignored the earlier signs and symptoms, and now it may be too late! You didn't take the Bang-Bang stage seriously. You didn't make the necessary changes in your life-style, behavior, and health habits. You may have continued to overstrain your body. Now, your major bodily organs are in jeopardy. Hospitalization, major surgery, intensive care, and prolonged convalescence are likely. Diagnoses such as stroke with partial paralysis, massive heart attack, cancer, major digestive disorders, and suicidal depression are all too common among nurses. Scary?—you bet!

The following quote from *The Self-Health Guide* (Kripalu Center for Holistic Health, Kripalu Publications, 1980, p. 23), describes the delicate interplay between the mind and the body:

> All stages of physical distress, from mere discomfort through severe pain, are simply messengers from prana [life breath or inner life force] with a single, simple purpose: to show us where we are going astray on the road of life and health, and to bring us back. They are like welcome lighthouses glimpsed through the fog, warning us to take our bearings and correct our course before we steer onto the rocks.
>
> Once we understand this, a change will happen in our attitude towards pain and sickness, health and life itself. We will become willing and able to respond to the warning signals that prana [our inner life force] puts out in the earliest stage, and so lead a life of prevention rather than cure.

This relationship between mind and body is something a nurse ultimately knows. We hope that you will choose to use this knowledge to your own advantage, tune yourself in to your early signs and symptoms, and help patients do the same. It's time to practice what you preach.

Now, stop a minute and look at yourself—at your early stress signs and symptoms. Figure 5-1 examines four categories of stress signals—emotional, physical, social, and performance-related. Take the time to look through the list and check off the signs and symptoms that relate to you. Several checks in any of the four categories

Figure 5-1. Taking Stock of Your Stress: Early Signs and Symptoms

Directions: Check off your signs and symptoms. Do this now and periodically to gain a better perspective on yourself.

Emotional

_____ Feeling irritable
_____ Feeling inadequate
_____ Having a tendency to cry easily
_____ Experiencing a loss of confidence
_____ Feeling cynical about your job
_____ Having a detached attitude
_____ Feeling stupid
_____ Feeling paranoid
_____ Constantly feeling rushed
_____ Feeling helpless

_____ Complaining
_____ Acting callous
_____ Feeling disillusioned
_____ Having a shortened attention span
_____ Feeling trapped and alone
_____ Feeling restless
_____ Feeling depressed
_____ Feeling like a failure
_____ Feeling overwhelmed
_____ Feeling unappreciated
_____ Never feeling finished
_____ Having outbursts of temper

_____ Feeling guilty
_____ Feeling bored
_____ Feeling worried
_____ Feeling scared
_____ Feeling anxious
_____ Being abrupt with people
_____ Feeling that catastrophes are impending
_____ Feeling impatient most of the time
_____ Experiencing recurring anger

Physical

_____ Having tight, tense muscles
_____ Having headaches
_____ Having insomnia
_____ Experiencing shallow breathing
_____ Having frequent colds
_____ Being overweight
_____ Drinking too much
_____ Having heart problems

_____ Having general aches and pains
_____ Feeling exhausted
_____ Experiencing hyperventilation
_____ Experiencing dizziness
_____ Having stomach distress
_____ Being out of shape

_____ Biting nails
_____ Feeling stiff
_____ Feeling run-down
_____ Having back pain
_____ Oversleeping
_____ Lacking energy
_____ Looking tired and washed out

Social

_____ Forgetting to smile
_____ Being preoccupied with work when off-duty
_____ Curtailing outside activities
_____ Having a change of personality for the worse
_____ Losing interest in activities once enjoyed
_____ Taking yourself too seriously

_____ Avoiding people
_____ Feeling distracted and detached
_____ Reneging on commitments
_____ Being unable to make decisions
_____ Feeling no sense of belonging at work
_____ Not initiating social times with friends

_____ Being unable to take a joke or be teased by others
_____ Seeing anything social as too much effort
_____ Making critical judgments of yourself and others

Continued on next page

Figure 5-1. (Continued)

Performance-Related

____ Living for the weekends or days off	____ Being late for work and meetings	____ Venting frustration on patients and coworkers
____ Absenteeism	____ Forgetting things	
____ Feeling inflexible in the face of change	____ Blaming others or finger-pointing	____ Making mistakes
____ Making a big deal out of small things	____ Taking longer and longer to get things done	____ Having difficulty receiving criticism
____ Having difficulty saying no		____ Procrastinating
	____ Having difficulty say-ing yes	____ Being unable to see alternatives in the face of problems
____ Having difficulty making decisions	____ Feeling performance is never good enough	____ Avoiding certain tasks
____ Not trusting your judgment or decisions		____ Making excuses

Several checks in any of the four categories indicate that your system is out of balance. Don't ignore these signs; take the necessary action immediately.

indicate that your system may be out of balance. If that is the case, it is time to take action now! Catch stress early.

The following section presents strategies for putting yourself back into balance and staying there.

Stress Skills and Strategies

Stress skills and strategies are actions you can take on your own behalf to attain the objectives in the following list:

- Get yourself unstuck from negative emotions and freed from the Self-Defeating Zone.
- Counteract the inevitable anxiety, frustrations, and tensions of your workday.
- Restore flexibility, adapt to change, and spring back from disappointments and setbacks.
- Build up strong reserves so that you have physical vitality and are equipped to fend off sickness.

These skills and strategies are divided into three categories:

1. Cognitive realignment
2. Practical wisdom
3. Relaxation techniques

Cognitive Realignment

Probably the most common contributor to stress is negative self-talk. Cognitive realignment deals directly with your inner monologue. You must reconstruct your usual thinking patterns so that they produce less stress for you. Chances are, you associate the word "realignment" with the concept of balance. That's exactly what it's about—putting yourself back in balance, so that stress works for you and not against you.

Positive Self-Talk: The Voice Within

When you think about it, the person you talk to the most in the course of a normal day is yourself. Your internal monologue can range from muttering about the weather to giving yourself encouragement during a challenging patient treatment.

What you say to yourself—your self-thoughts—has a dramatic impact on your stress level. Self-thoughts can create confidence or anxiety, courage or fear, love or hate. That voice within can be your best friend or your own worst enemy. It's your choice. Are you ready to say goodbye to negative self-talks and hello to positive self-talks? Here's how:

1. **Acknowledgment:** Admit to yourself that you do indeed engage in "negative self-talk."

   I, _____, do engage in "negative self-talk."
2. **Spotlighting negativism:** Each time you're feeling a negative emotion (that is, disorganization, frustration, anger, depression, crankiness, helplessness, indecisiveness, fear, irritability, withdrawal, and so on), turn on your internal flashlight and spotlight the negative self-talk that's attached to your feeling.
3. **Cognitive realignment:** Replace the negative thought with a positive one.

   "I can't" becomes "I can."
   "I don't" becomes "I do."
   "I'll try" becomes "I will."

Antidote to Anger

Do you accept anger as part of your life? Have you ever said, "I can't help it . . . I've got a short fuse"? Or, "I'm only human." Or, better yet, "If I don't express it, then I'll keep it inside and get an ulcer." Although suppressing your anger is not healthy, it would certainly be healthier to feel angry less often.

You can implement two plans:

1. **The Coping Plan,** for expressing anger and reducing its negative effects
2. **The Anger Elimination Plan,** for choosing to feel less anger in your life

The Coping Plan: Imagine that this morning has been a disaster. The support services are a joke. Your patients are sicker than you've expected and are very dependent. The doctor is nowhere to be found; the level of staffing is bordering on unsafe; and, to top it off, you've just found out that the nurse who promised to work for you, so that you could be home on your daughter's birthday, is backing out with a flimsy excuse.

Instead of fuming about your problems and dwelling on what you'd like to call your coworker, try this first:

- **Stop** and admit, "I'm angry!"
- **Quickly, take your anger temperature.** (Is it 110 degrees or 98.6 degrees?) If you rate your level of anger high on the scale of 98.6 to 110, you can reduce your anger temperature automatically by recognizing that you're in the danger zone. That awareness will shock you into a position of gaining greater control of your emotions.
- **Try one of these alternatives:**
  Option 1: Get your anger out. Let it come out your arm and onto paper! Ventilate your anger by writing about it. Set aside a notebook in a handy place—at work, at home, or both—or just carry a small tablet in your uniform pocket. When anger grabs you, pick up a pen and write nonstop for 3 minutes. Don't think about what to say. Pay no attention to spelling, grammar, or punctuation. Just let your feelings spill out on paper. If 3 minutes is not enough, keep writing until you feel a sense of release. Writing helps you clear the air, so that you can regain your perspective and see your next action step more clearly. Now, create a burial ceremony. Take your pages of angry outpourings. Rip them up. Destroy them. You sure don't want them lingering around! Besides, the symbolic act of burying them can help purge the stress from your system and restore your balance more quickly.
  Option 2: Physically vent your anger. Physical action can be a good release. Go for a fast-paced walk on your break or lunch hour. If you're going home, clean out a cluttered closet, wash the car, or jog your anger away. You'll reduce stress and build productive energy.

The Anger Elimination Plan: Your anger and the way you express and handle it may be an established habit, but you still have a choice. You can learn alternative behavior. You can eliminate anger before it begins. If you can prevent it, you don't have to bother coping with it.

As is the case with other emotions, anger is the result of your thoughts. So, let's consider how to realign the thinking associated with anger. Here are tips on how to think differently and, as a result, rid yourself of this emotion that, ultimately, can hurt you:

- **Deal with reality.** People will do things in ways you won't like. Things will inevitably not go in the direction you may want or expect. By denying this reality, you deny other people the right to be who they are. You resist the flow of life, which you can't control anyway. Annoyances, disappointments, curveballs, the unexpected—that's all part of life. The probability that you'll change it is highly unlikely. So, instead of choosing anger, you can reframe your thoughts about others and accept that they have a right to be different from what you expect or want. The key to this new mind-set is recognition that you might not like it, *but you don't have to get angry about it.* Let's look at new anger-free thoughts:
  —She may be a jerk, but I don't have to let her actions upset me.
  —It's true that I look bad, even though he caused the problem. The solution within my control is to drop a note of apology. Meanwhile, I'm choosing to be free of anger because it only hurts me—no one else.
  —I can stop his behavior from affecting me. My getting angry isn't going to change him, so why waste my good energy?
- **Postpone anger.** You can learn to control your anger through brief postponements—15 seconds, 30 seconds (the old count-to-10 trick). Then, keep extending the intervals. With patience, you can learn to do away with anger altogether by rewiring your response through steady, consistent postponement.
- **Fake it, if you need to.** If anger, at times, seems to get you the results you want, fake it. Raise your voice and look stern (for example, alerting your child to a dangerous situation), but don't set off your stress alarm and experience all the physical wear and tear.
- **Switch from anger to dislike.** In your mind's eye, picture a switch that reads "dislike" and another that reads "anger." Turn off the "anger switch" and turn on the "dislike switch." You can *dislike* something *but* choose not to be angry about it.

- **Hire a coach.** Ask a coworker you trust to be your anger coach. Ask your coach to signal you each time you show signs of anger. Agree ahead of time on a signal. Once you get the signal, switch to the postponement technique.
- **Play "Monday-morning quarterback."** You fumbled or handled a situation badly. Then you had an angry outburst. You can see that after the fact. Fine. It's valuable learning. Grab a friend and tell the friend where you slipped up and what you want to think or do differently next time. By making this a public commitment, you put yourself back on the right track with new momentum.
- **Drop expectations of others.** When you let go of your image of what others should be and what they should do, you can let go of your anger.
- **Value your health.** If you do, you won't even consider disabling yourself with self-destructive anger.

Overcoming Guilt

One of the greatest sources of stress reported by nurses is the guilt that builds from the discrepancy between the "ideal" and the "real." You know the care and attention patients need and deserve. You are also well aware of the reality of what "staffing" and "the system" actually allow. Piles of guilt can accumulate in the gap between the ideal and the real. The experience of guilt results from awareness of that gap.

Too often, your mind dwells on all the things you couldn't get to, everything that was left undone, and what you had to let go of because there just wasn't time. This is when you wake up out of a sound sleep startled, remembering what you forgot—a medication error, leaving a patient on the bedpan. Long after your shift is over, feelings linger about the tension you might have conveyed to patients, and about times when you were abrupt with your patients at work and with your family at home.

A snowball of guilt turns into an avalanche of self-recrimination. Experiencing guilt, you focus on a past event and feel anxiety and regret. The result: you rob your present moment of happiness, effectiveness, and personal well-being.

As a nurse, you get a double dose of guilt—one dose from ordinary human shortcomings, another from being a health care professional who is supposed to be all things to all people and provide "total care." Somehow, our society has linked caring to a sense of inadequacy or guilt over shortcomings. Do you think you're a bad nurse if you don't feel guilt most of the time?

Guilt is a prizewinning waster of your emotional energy. Usually, it serves no useful purpose. You're occupying your present moment with thoughts about a past event or a missed opportunity that no amount of guilt can change. Guilt-induced anxiety ranges from slight upset to deep depression.

What can you do? The first step in overcoming guilt is to distinguish between guilt and learning from your mistakes. If you are learning from your past to avoid future mistakes, this is not guilt. *Guilt is when you don't act in the present moment because you're caught up in what happened to you yesterday.* For example:

- You avoid a certain patient's room today because you didn't stop in as you promised yesterday.
- You don't ask for help with a specific clinical procedure because you think you should have learned it in a recent mandatory in-service.

Not only is guilt a waste of energy and time, it sets you back even further each time you dwell on it. Consider the example of feeling guilty about cheating on your diet. You eat one piece of cake and you feel bad for two days for having been weak. Your self-reproach trip sends you further into the counterproductive behavior you're trying to overcome. Instead of getting back on course with your diet, you disable yourself by thinking, "What's the use? I don't have the discipline to diet; I'm a lazy slob." And, in all probability, you eat more.

Get a handle on your guilt and conquer it bit by bit. Here's how:

- **Clearly identify guilt by honestly answering your own question.** "Is this bad feeling I'm having related to guilt? Do I feel guilty about something? If so, what?"
- **Ask a second-level question.** "Is it logical and rational for me to feel guilty? Is this feeling of guilt useful in any way? Is this feeling of guilt enabling or disabling my performance?"

  To help you answer this, remember the distinction made earlier. If your response spurs you to activity, recognize that you're learning from your past, and do not label it as guilt. If the feeling immobilizes you, causes you sadness, anxiety, tension, or fear, and makes you want to pull back or withdraw from people, you need to admit to the pain you're inflicting on yourself and choose not to continue doing that! Be gentle with yourself; forgive yourself!

- **Nurture the thought that "the past is history."** You can't relive it or change it. It's over and gone. All the guilt you can muster will not make the past different. Burn this thought into your brain. Affirmation: "My feelings of guilt will never undo the past, nor will they help me to be the best person I can be right now."
- **Direct energy into working on what, by being stuck on guilt, you're avoiding in the present.** Remember the example of the procedure you needed help with? Instead of spinning your wheels with guilt, you could tackle the need to feel more competent as an educational adventure. Set up a refresher with a friend; read whatever materials you can find, and make yourself an expert in this medical area.
- **Keep a running tab of your guilty moments.** Write them down with whens, whys, and whos. You might gain insight into your particular patterns and be better able to see what you're avoiding in the present.
- **Turn off the guilt faucet.** So often, after a guilt-inducing event, you replay over and over in your mind how terrible you feel about it. This is when you need to terminate the guilty thoughts, literally making a decision to bury the past.

Overcoming Worry

Worry and guilt are perhaps the two most common forms of distress for nurses. Whether you're stuck on guilt about yesterday or polluting tomorrow with worry, the result is the same: You're throwing away your energy for the present.

To overcome worry, replace it with action planning. When you redirect your energy to planning for the future, you take control. Let's look more closely at some of the underlying reasons why people invest in worry:

- **You avoid and escape what threatens you about "now."** *Example:* I'm so worried about tomorrow because of the predicted bad weather that I can't concentrate on writing this quality assurance report.
- **You avoid taking a risk by busying yourself with worry.** Then you cite worry as the reason for your inaction. *Example:* "How can I take an exercise class when I'm constantly worried about whether my teenage children are safe at home?"
- **You can regard yourself as a more caring, responsible person by worrying.** Worry proves you are a good, caring nurse, a good parent, a good friend.

Example: "I had indigestion all night worrying about Mr. Smith and his condition."

- **Worry supports you in being lazy.** A worrier sits and ponders things, while a doer is up and moving.
  Example: "I'd better say no. Go ahead without me. I've been worried about my parents. Even though they won't be here for a few days, I'm scared that something will happen to them along the way. You know all the crazy things that have been happening with airplanes lately."
- **Worry is a great justification for undisciplined behavior,** such as overeating or not exercising.
  Example: "I've gained so much weight. I've been so worried about John and his grades that I can't help it."

Think for a few minutes about whether the payoffs indicated above are worth the stressfulness of the worry involved. If you conclude that you want to worry less, consider these devices for eliminating or at least reducing worry.

Take action. The best remedy for worry is action. Keep yourself moving. Tackle that task, make that call, write that memo, fold those clothes. When you're occupied and engaged in an activity, you focus your mind on that activity, and worry subsides.

Confront your motive. Ask yourself a direct question that uncovers your underlying motivation for worrying. Example: "What am I avoiding right now by falling into the trap of worrying?" Then plow ahead and tackle whatever you're avoiding. Force a breakthrough.

Create a specific time for worrying. Set aside worry times. Select 10-minute intervals at the beginning or end of the day. Fill these designated periods with fuming and fretting about every conceivable disaster you can think of. Jam them into one of these two time slots. The challenge is to make all other time worry-free. If a worried thought enters your head, postpone it until your next worry period. You can do this by taking charge of your thoughts.

Take stock of your past worries. On a clean piece of paper, jot down everything you worried about yesterday, last week, last month, and even last year. Try to think of worries that were resolved as well as those that weren't. Then, taking each item at a time, ask yourself the following questions:

1. Did worrying itself change anything?
2. Did what I worried would happen actually happen?
3. Did the event I worried about turn out to be a major catastrophe?
4. Did the event turn out to be insignificant?
5. Did the event turn out to be positive?

You can use this list and your responses to draw conclusions about the cost-effectiveness of worrying. That is, do the benefits of worrying justify the time and energy directed toward it? Chances are, you'll find they don't, and you'll choose to redirect your energies toward positive, benefits-producing activities.

Embrace the mind-set of the half-full glass. Look at a glass with water up to its midpoint. Is it half empty or half full? If your immediate response is "half empty," chances are that you have a tendency to view things with a pessimistic eye. Do you have a positive or negative attitude? Which list in figure 5-2 describes your mind-set best?

A negative mind-set burns your energy. A positive mind-set generates energy. If you feed your unconscious with negative messages, you will create your own negative reality. For example, if you beat yourself up about what you can't get done, your thoughts trigger an overwhelmed feeling. You muddle your mind, then make a mistake or misjudge an important decision. As a result, you feel bad, you fall further behind, you get increasingly anxious. It becomes a vicious cycle or self-fulfilling prophecy; that is, what you expect is what you get. As you work to convince yourself of your limitations, you ensure that they will, in fact, be yours. On the other hand, if you concentrate on your capabilities, you generate productive energy, you become more efficient, and your reality becomes more positive.

Shift into neutral. Instead of reacting with good or bad, right or wrong, judgment, evaluation, and criticism, shift your mind into neutral for a welcome change. Neutrality is an easygoing, mellow, stress-free position. It's within your power to select the option of neutrality. This is not the mind-set of a lazy person. On the contrary, it is a creative reaction to events that you cannot control. Rather than waste energy being angry or wishing things were different, you do the best you can under the circumstances. For example: You find that the linen is delayed until 11 a.m. Instead of getting angry or frustrated, do what you can with what you have until 11:00. Or, at the end of the day, you wish you had accomplished more. Take stock and see what you did accomplish and be understanding of your

Figure 5-2. Negative Focus versus Positive Focus

Negative Focus	Positive Focus
• What's not working	• What *is* working
• What's bad about the day	• What's good about the day
• What you're dreading	• What you're looking forward to
• The patients who are nasty and miserable	• The patients who are grateful and wonderful

limitations. Decide to feel good about what you accomplished. It may be that you could have done more; but then, you also could have done a lot less!

Stop setting yourself up for failure. A major source of stress for many nurses is the unrealistic expectations they set up for themselves. Although idealism and striving for excellence are certainly vital to high-quality patient care, you can carry these too far. Much stress comes from self-imposed demands and the self-inflicted pressure to be the perfect nurse. To reduce stress from self-imposed unrealistic expectations, try these approaches:

- **If you tend to be an overachiever, knock your expectations down two notches before you begin your day.** This will relieve you immediately and ensure a greater possibility of success.

- **On days when your unit is short-staffed, take immediate stock of reality.** Plug in to an inner dialogue that supports you and keeps your own self-expectations in check. Tell yourself, "I can't beat myself up because I can't do it all. I'll do what I can and do it with joy in my heart."

- **Be honest with yourself about what's doable.** Do you ever fool yourself about what you can accomplish in a day or what you can do and be for people? If so, you inflict stress unnecessarily on yourself. Think about your expectations. Ask yourself, "From my past experience, is all of this doable, or am I being unrealistic?" For example, the next time someone asks you when they can have your report, don't say "20 minutes" just because you think that's what they want to hear, if you know realistically that it will take 40 minutes.

Mental rehearsal. You've been reading a lot about what not to say to yourself. The four-step process that follows describes what you can and should say to yourself. Do you remember when you learned to ride a bike or drive a car? Chances are, you talked to yourself, step-by-step, even out loud. Talking to yourself helped you get through the learning stages of mastering these new skills. The same technique helps people deal with stressful situations.

The following four coaching statements are particularly powerful: initiation, line-up-your-ducks, positive pep, and pat-on-the-back statements:

- **"Initiation" statements.** When you're gearing up for an encounter, say out loud a rational statement that instills confidence.
  Example: "OK, Jackie. You can handle Dr. Blakely just fine. Your concern about Mrs. Root is legitimate, and you have the

ability to be clear and to the point. You're ready. All you have to do is stay centered and calm."

- **"Line-up-your-ducks" statements.** Outline, step-by-step, what you need to do and say in order to make your transaction successful.
  Example: "I need to say 'Good morning, Dr. Blakely' in a professional manner—OK, I did it . . . that was great. Now I need to tell her in one sentence what my concerns are, turning to the patient's input/output record in the medical chart. OK, that's done. Now, I need to ask her opinion and, last, get an order for an additional medication. Bingo! I did it."
- **"Positive pep" statements.** Here, you support yourself with reassuring messages, messages that calm you and bolster your courage and confidence.
  Example: "You work extremely well with people. Remember, just stay calm, speak directly, and look right at the patient. You're a very competent nurse. Trust yourself. Don't be intimidated."
- **"Pat-on-the-back" statements.** You completed your task or encounter. Congratulate yourself. Bask in the satisfaction.
  Example: "You did it, and it went just fine. You handled it like a pro. You were cool and calm, and you spoke out for what you believed was right. Good job!"

Use these four coaching statements to rehearse before a stressful event or interaction and to enable and energize yourself during and after the event or the interaction itself.

Another technique that can be used is known as *relabeling the event.* Often, when circumstances don't work out as planned, you find yourself feeling frustrated, tense, and irritable. Instead of dwelling in the Self-Defeating Zone, you can relabel or rename the event. This skill enables you to find the promise or opportunity in the problem at hand. Relabeling involves taking negative circumstances and literally flipping them around in your mind so that you focus on the brighter side—on the side of opportunity. The following examples illustrate this technique:

- **Example 1:** You drive to the mall and you want to park close, but there's no nearby spot.
  Relabel: "No spot. But this is a chance to get some exercise, and the fresh air will do me good."
- **Example 2:** You have an evening out planned with two close friends, and at the last minute, one of them cancels. You're disappointed.

Relabel: "Although I'll miss seeing Janet, it will be a chance to be with Marsha. This quality time with Marsha will be an opportunity."

Example 3: You have been asked to change your usual lunch hour from 12 to 1. You're annoyed.

Relabel: "The cafeteria will be a lot less crowded, and it will give me a chance to sit with new folks. Besides, the afternoon will go faster."

Relabeling is a trump card in stress management. It involves finding the positive value in whatever way the cards fall. And it pays off—over and over!

Practical Wisdom

"We make our habits and then our habits make us." Sound familiar? Most of us are creatures of habit. Some of these habits are good—they enhance our life. But others are not so good. In fact, some habits can be destructive—and these, of course, do not enhance our lives. Our habits are learned, and consciously or unconsciously we select which habits to call our own. This selection, by and large, is made on the basis of our personal values. This section talks about your values and the commitments you make, keep, and don't keep that reflect your value system.

Live and Work by Your Values

Your values influence your choices and decisions at work, and they determine what is worth getting upset about, where your priorities are, how you wish to spend your time, and what is important to fight for. If you constantly feel unwelcome stress, it's time for values clarification and a concerted effort to check the "fit" between your values and the way you really spend your time.

Figure 5-3 presents a list of work-related values. From the list, select five items that you value most in your work life. Add your own if you wish. Then, note the values of work that cause you the most stress.

Now complete figure 5-4 by looking over the five values you've checked in the previous figure. List and rank order these values and record the corresponding stress level next to each one. Next, construct a one-minute action plan by asking yourself the following question: "What do I need to do to put my values back into balance? What trade-offs am I willing to make? Where do I want to begin?"

Note: Be as concrete and specific as you can be. Give yourself a deadline by which you intend to do something; for example, speak

Figure 5-3. Work Values and Related Stress Levels

Directions: Check off on the line at the left the five values below that are most important to you. What is your stress level in relation to each? On the line at the right of each value, rate your stress level in relation to that work value.

Work Value	Stress Level (on a scale of 1 to 10; 10 is high)
_____ Quality of patient care	_____
_____ Honest feedback	_____
_____ Ethical medical practice	_____
_____ Pleasant work environment	_____
_____ Holistic approach to nursing	_____
_____ Interdepartmental cooperation	_____
_____ Camaraderie	_____
_____ Financial compensation	_____
_____ Medical technology	_____
_____ Support and involvement of patients' families	_____
_____ Bedside care	_____
_____ Working with physicians as colleagues	_____
_____ Career advancement	_____
_____ Health benefits	_____
_____ Good hours	_____
_____ Continuing education	_____
_____ Peer support	_____
_____ Satisfaction/renewal	_____
_____ Effective communication with boss	_____
_____ Developing my talent	_____
_____ Fun and leisure	_____
_____ Other	_____

Figure 5-4. The One-Minute Action Plan

The Five Values Most Important to Me on the Job	Stress Level (1-10)	One-Minute Action Plan
1. _____	_____	_____
2. _____	_____	_____
3. _____	_____	_____
4. _____	_____	_____
5. _____	_____	_____

to Dr. Miserable with "Hello. How are you?" for the next five days, starting tomorrow. The following examples illustrate:

- **Example 1:** Let's say you chose *honest feedback* as a most important value, and the stress level is an 8. A one-minute action might be to ask two colleagues to sit down and listen to you do your own self-assessment of strengths and weaknesses on the job. Ask them to add their input by such and such a date. If you decide to get brave, you can initiate the same exercise with your boss, also putting a deadline to it. Remember, if feedback is important, and you're not getting enough, then you need to do the asking.
- **Example 2:** You chose *pleasant work environment* as a most important value (stress level is a 9). Your one-minute action plan might be to make a commitment not to allow yourself to get dragged into the complaining on the unit or to join in the moaning and groaning for the next three days.

Make a Commitment and Follow Through

As commitments to these one-minute action plans fall by the way-side, people tend to feel stress and inadequacy. If you're wondering why your life lacks accomplishment, chances are, *you haven't made a serious commitment to making things happen.* Reduce the stress of inaction and give yourself the gusto to get where you want to go and be all you want to be. Follow these steps:

- **Make conscious, not half-baked, commitments.** Half-baked commitments produce stress. When you're at a cross-road, stop and consider these questions:
  —How important is this to me?
  —How much am I willing to do or to sacrifice to make it happen?
  —Am I ready to make a serious commitment to making it happen, or will my dedication fizzle?
  —Will I honestly use my full potential to honor this commitment?
- **Write down your commitments.** Documenting your commitments makes them more concrete and builds momentum toward making them a reality.
- **Make your commitment public.** Post it. Tell a coworker, friend, or loved one what you want to do—and will do. Ask for their support and assistance. Arrange times to check in with them, so they can help you monitor your progress. Share your ups and downs. By making your commitment public, you establish accountability and support for yourself.

- **Make fewer agreements, and keep the ones you make.** If you are like most people, you agree to do things without first thinking carefully about what the commitment entails. When you don't follow through, you end up feeling overwhelmed, guilty, and frustrated. Stop! Be more selective and decide that the agreements you do make are ones you are going to honor.
- **Let people know if you can't fulfill an agreement.** Sometimes people procrastinate and avoid fulfilling commitments until it's too late to honor them. This is the quintessential stress-producing situation. If you see a problem ahead, blow the whistle early. Let people know where you are and why. Offer an alternative. Renegotiate the deadline or consider other options for getting it done.
- **Acquire time-management skills.** Proper time management is a stress-crippler. Watch your language. "If only I had time." "There is just too much to do and not enough time." "I'll never get finished." Is this language part of your litany? Talking about time robs you of time and ends up making you more anxious and less effective. Take time to plan your day before you begin it. This will save you time and stress. Write out your plan on a small notepad. For example:
  —Arrange your duties in the most efficient order (that is, do errands all at once; lump phone calls together; call when you are most likely to reach people; shop at the least hectic times).
  —Organize your tasks in priority order.
  —Write down a "to do" list that is doable. It is stressful to keep such lists in your head.
  —Handle each piece of paper only once.
  —Ask yourself frequently, "Is this the best use of my time right now?"
- **Unclock yourself.** When you are off duty, take off your watch and enjoy getting in touch with your natural rhythm.
- **Live and work by the slogan "Do it now."** If a patient wants a drink of water, do it now instead of saying to yourself that you'll get back to her. The more you pile up for later, the more stress you'll feel and the more you'll forget. You'll be overloading your circuit.
- **Express your feelings about starting on time.** When scheduling a meeting or lunch date, don't hesitate to let people know your time parameters. Use simple statements like, "My time is tight today; I only have the hour. Can we cover what we need to do?" Not only does the other person now

know your limits, but you have also stressed the need to be prompt.

- **Give patients realistic time estimates.** How often do you promise to "be back in a minute"? Although it comforts patients to hear how long you'll be, it agitates them when your time estimate creates false expectations. Give patients realistic time estimates while acknowledging their needs. Example: "I know how important it is to you to get your diet straightened out; I'll be sure to call the dietician before 3:00 p.m.," or, "I know you've been waiting patiently. It will be 15 minutes more."

Relaxation Techniques

In the active and demanding world of nursing, it's easy to forget that periods of relaxation and rest are as crucial to your well-being as the air you breathe. Relaxation is not something you need only when you're tense or unoccupied. Relaxation is an attitude—a way of working—a state of mind that allows ease, grace, and dignity. Once you learn to work in a relaxed, alert state, you have the ability to greatly diminish tension and stress. When you operate from a mental and physical position of relaxation, you become a sponge, drawing in new energy, freedom, and stability.

Nurses are now involved in more high-stress situations than ever before. Since an estimated 80 percent of illness is believed to be stress-related, your life literally depends on learning to alleviate or prevent tension.

Earlier, this book examined "mental tools" for stress management. Now it's time to explore physical relaxation techniques that elevate your energy and insulate you from the general wear and tear of today's working conditions.

Breathing

Breathing has a profound effect on our ability to release tension, avoid stress, and relax. How aware are you of the manner of your breathing at any given moment? The act of breathing is so automatic that we completely underutilize its life-giving capabilities.

The following passage, from *The Self-Health Guide* (Kripalu Center for Holistic Health, Kripalu Publications, 1980, p. 62) is an excellent description of "how to breathe." You'd be surprised how many of us are breathing improperly. Try this technique:

> Imagine that you have a balloon inside and as you inhale you are slowly inflating it, causing the abdominal area to slowly swell. Feel your diaphragm being pushed down and relaxing.

Breathe out slowly through your nose as you pull your abdominal muscles in, without straining, so that you press all of the air out of your lungs. Continue breathing in as the abdomen rises and out as it falls, until you've established a natural rhythm.

Hint: Place your hands on your abdomen, just above the navel, with fingertips pointing towards each other and just touching. If you are breathing correctly, as you inhale your hands will rise with your abdomen and your fingertips will separate. As you exhale, they will touch again.

Proper breathing, alone or in combination with other relaxation exercises such as progressive muscle relaxation and visualization techniques, reduces anxiety before and during stressful situations. Relaxation exercises have an immediate calming effect and instill a sense of balance and control. Consider practicing a relaxation skill several times a day. You can do it without anyone even noticing, and you don't have to stop your activities. After practicing conscious breathing, it will become a practically automatic tension reducer.

Progressive Relaxation

Through progressive relaxation, you can become aware of your level of tension and relaxation, discover which muscle groups hold your tension, and learn to relax all of these major muscle groups. Start by doing relaxation exercises in a quiet, comfortable place. Recline or stretch out on the floor. Once you get the hang of it, you'll be able to do parts of the exercises quickly at your work station. Try this sampling of exercises (excerpted from *The Self-Health Guide* published by Kripalu Publications):

- **Regulate your breath.** Begin to take long, deep, and uniform breaths, gradually slowing down the rate of your breathing. By slowing your breathing tempo to the rate of approximately three heartbeats each inhalation, five to each exhalation, your body and mind will begin to relax and slow down. Continue with this breathing pattern until you have sunk deeply into relaxation.
- **Progressively relax each muscle.** As you continue with deep breathing, begin to consciously relax your muscles. Mentally traveling through your body, tell each part to relax, one by one, from the toes to the top of your head. With each exhalation, feel as if you are letting go, breathing out tiredness, stress, tension from that body part. With each inhalation, feel yourself breathing in relaxation.

Relax your body parts in this order: feet, ankles, calves, knees, thighs, hips, abdominal muscles, then the muscles of the back, chest, shoulders, arms, and hands. Relax your neck and skull. Then relax your face. Drop any tensions that surround the eyes, and let all facial expressions fall away. Relax your forehead and the sides of your face. Allow your jaw to sag slightly, parting your lips, and relax.

- **Calm your nervous system.** When your muscles and organs have become relaxed, begin to consciously relax your nerves. Try to discover where the inner pockets of tension lie within your body. As they reveal themselves to your inner gaze, visualize the incoming breath dissolving these buried tensions. Expel their last vestiges with each exhalation. Feel that your tired and overworked nervous channels are closing down, that communication between your brain and nerve centers is being temporarily suspended. Let go; imagine your mind as a clear blue sky with thoughts as slowly floating clouds. Feel your body grow heavier and heavier as it sinks into the floor.

- **Calm your mind; let go.** Now send your mind as far as it can go from your everyday life. Leave your anxieties and worries, your obligations and responsibilities. Create a strong mental image of a place where you are completely free, completely at peace. Perhaps you will visualize a sunny beach or a silent garden. Retreat into this, your personal sanctuary, leaving only your body lying on the floor. Be completely in your imagined retreat, in a state devoid of all fears for the future and all regrets over the past. Secure in the knowledge that you are at home within yourself, allow your conscious mind to drift into a state of blankness. You'll feel restored!

- **Gently come back.** Stay in this state for as long as you wish. When your consciousness begins to return to your body, do not sit up right away. Instead, linger in the twilight state for a short time, gently stretching your body in the way that feels most natural for you. After a few minutes open your eyes and slowly sit up.

  (*Note:* You can ask someone to read the preceding instructions to you, or you can put them on a tape so they're handy when you need them.)

Visualization

Visualization is a powerful relaxation tool. It's a form of daydreaming that you can use to help yourself relax and renew. Visualization works like this:

Close your eyes and take deep, tension-releasing breaths. Imagine a specific scene that would offer peaceful relaxation, such as lying on the grass in a quiet park. Continue to develop the scene. Imagine the fresh smell of grass and flowers, the sound of birds singing softly in the trees, the warmth of the sun on your face, a gentle breeze caressing your skin . . . .

If you concentrate on the scene, you will begin to feel as relaxed as you would if you were really lying on the grass.

You can use visualization, like breathing exercises, at work when you're feeling tired and tense. During your break, or whenever you have a few free minutes, seek a quiet place (hospital chapels or reading rooms are great) and relax into a soothing visualization.

Use the following imagery, or experiment to find the fantasy that works best for you:

1. **You're lying on the beach, warm under the sun.** The sand feels nice and soft beneath you. You're calm and relaxed, almost falling asleep. You can hear the waves rolling in gently. You feel so comfortable . . . .
2. **You are walking slowly through a beautiful green forest.** You can hear only the sounds of the birds in the distance. It is very quiet here, and you continue to walk slowly and quietly, enjoying the calm and peacefulness. It is a warm day, but the forest is slightly cool, making you feel very comfortable, just the right temperature. You have the forest all to yourself with nothing to disturb you, just feeling good, feeling calm and relaxed.
3. **You are sitting on a bank at the side of a lake.** The water is very still and quite clear. The lake is flat and shiny. If you look into the distance you can see the water sparkling from the sun shining on it. It is very comfortable where you're sitting. You find it so easy to relax and just gaze out at the lake.

Meditation

Because peace of mind comes from within, not from material objects or external stimulation, you can cultivate it. The goal is to be calm, focus your restless mind, and achieve a sense of peaceful coexistence with the physical world. If possible, take 20 minutes of every day to be alone in a quiet place. Concentrate on your breath, practicing the breathing technique described in the previous section. Let your thoughts come and go without concern or attachment. Just keep your mind focused on your abdomen as it rises and falls with each inhalation and exhalation of breath. Soon your mind will become quiet, and your body will relax.

Massage

As nurses, you know better than most the benefit of therapeutic touch. In ancient times, the Greeks, the Romans, and the Egyptians used massage to relieve pain and restore the body. It still works!

Throughout your days as nurses, you are constantly exposed to tension-provoking situations. When your mind is stressed, your brain releases signals to your body—headache, stiff neck, back pain, jaw clenching, facial tension. Unless you release the tension, your body remains "electrified" with tension and anxiety. Over the years, this unreleased tension mounts, resulting in more health complications.

Generally, tension builds and strikes a specific part of your body recurrently—lower back pain or migraine headaches. These patterns of tension can block energy, like a garden hose tangled in one spot so the water can't rush through. Massage works to "rub out" or unblock these centers of tension.

Massage has specific therapeutic benefits. In physiological terms, what happens in the course of a thorough, therapeutic, deep body massage is this:

- The circulation improves as the blood vessels dilate from the warmth of friction.
- Wastes and toxins are released and eliminated from the tense muscles by the pressure.
- Improved circulation and relaxation of the muscle fibers increase the flow of nutrients to the muscles.

In every community, at health clubs, community centers, and health centers, massage services exist. Consider this a gift to yourself. Better yet, make it a steady diet. *The point is to take the time to master at least one relaxation technique, so that you feel equipped to relax regularly and when you're in tough circumstances.*

Summary

In this chapter we've examined stress, where it comes from and what it can do to your body as well as to your motivation and success. We've talked about the four stages of stress, as well as strategies for combating stress through cognitive realignment, attention to your values, and relaxation techniques. We've demonstrated that stress is not only damaging to your physical health but also interferes with effective job performance and with your personal happiness.

Stress, worry, guilt, unfulfilled commitments—all of these undermine your well-being and your ability to function at peak performance as a nurse. But the good news is that you can *choose* to give them up—to free yourself of the shackles of stress and even to make mild stress work for you, rather than against you.

We hope that the exercises in this chapter have given you food for thought and that you will begin to be consciously aware of the stresses that bog you down. Identifying the sources of stress is the first step toward finding a path out of the quagmire of stress, worry, and guilt and stepping into the sunshine of serene and successful living and working.

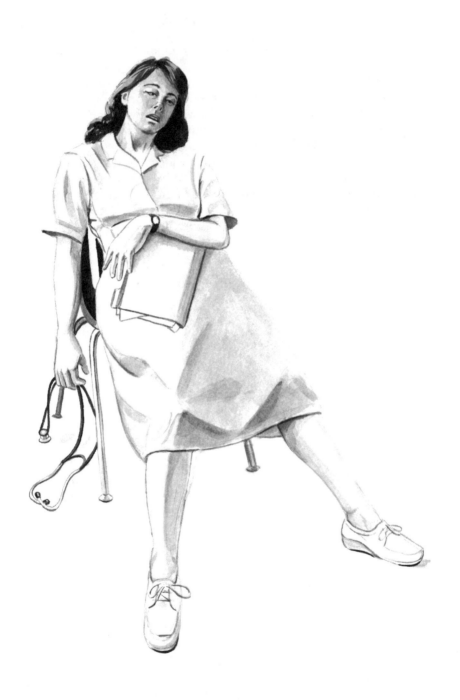

Chapter 6

Energy

This chapter will explore this concept: *The quality of energy we put into our work determines the benefits we gain from our work.* If we use our energy to its fullest, we can transform our work lives. Therefore, it is most important for nurses to find the most effective use of energy, not to waste a drop, and to take advantage of each moment of working time.

The key to free-flowing energy is relaxation in everything you do. Yes! We're advocating relaxation on the job! But how can nurses be relaxed at work? Relaxation doesn't mean sitting in the middle of the unit in a lounge chair with your sunglasses on and sipping a glass of iced tea. Hardly. Relaxation at work means working without carrying all the tension. It's an attitude—a way of being. Tension blocks the flow of energy. When our energy is not free to move, we get irritable, frustrated, impatient, tired, and overwhelmed.

Think about all the nurses you've worked with. Now think of just one person whom you would describe as having the ability to work relaxed. Did you come up with someone? Chances are that you did, because those relaxed people are out there. But isn't it inevitable that we should feel tired by the end of the shift and exhausted by the end of the work week? After all, look at all we do as nurses. Look at how hard we're working. Isn't it a given that all your energy would be spent at the end of an incredibly demanding day? Not necessarily.

Think of people whose energy seems boundless, who are in high-pressured, challenging positions, and yet they go, go, go and give, give, give . . . and never seem to tire. What's their secret?

Loving what you do helps. However, even in the most gratifying professions like nursing, stress and tension can pile up and destroy the good feelings you have. The secret is conservation of energy.

Conservation of energy entails two objectives:

- Consciously spending the energy we have wisely, not throwing it away or wasting it
- Learning to take in more than the average amount of life-giving energy

Ways of Redirecting Your Energy

Change Your Attitude toward Work

A great deal of our energy is tied up in the attitudes we have about our work. Negative work attitudes can cause us to experience our work day as tiring or tension-producing.

Do you see work as a necessary evil? Do you consider it nothing more than a means to an end? Do you see work as a duty that cannot be avoided—a time-consuming part of our lives? Do you expect to dislike your work? It's not hard to imagine that if any one of the above is a true underlying attitude of yours, you would be experiencing low energy and tons of tension. Just reading them is a downer, let alone living them week after week.

A redefinition of the meaning of work may be helpful. Try redefining your own concept of work. What definition do you *want* to live with? Once you've reworked your definition, it can direct your attitudes and actions as you work. An example of a positive definition of work is: "My work is the creative expression of my mind, body, and soul and a pathway to make my life joyful, fulfilling, and productive." Now imagine if you lived and worked by that definition how much more energy-filled and motivating your day as a nurse would be.

Our attitudes that flow from our own definitions of work greatly influence the energy we bring to our work. Our attitudes decree how much satisfaction, pleasure, and fulfillment we derive from our jobs.

Take a moment or two to write a healthy, reasonable, and energy-releasing definition of work.

My definition of work is: _____

_____

Don't Be Ruled by Expectations

Probably the most common tension-producing and energy-draining attitudes in nursing—and yet ones we are least aware of—are the expectations we bring to our jobs. We are constantly formulating expectations without realizing it. We expect to get our work finished in a certain amount of time, with the total cooperation of other people. We expect all the ancillary departments with which nursing interfaces to run smoothly, with no hitches. We expect praise or we expect blame, we expect appreciation or criticism. Whether it's good or bad, we're always expecting. Whether our expectations are optimistic or pessimistic, we continue anticipating the outcome: the way it should go, the way we expect it to be. It's so automatic we do it unconsciously.

Anticipation of the outcome of events can be a source of chronic tension in itself. One step in relieving this tension is to stop anticipating outcomes and to let go of expectations—or at least become aware of them and give your mind permission to be less of a judge and jury. We are not suggesting that you drop all performance expectations. Conforming to expectations is vital to the running of the hospital. Dietary, for example, cannot show up any time they feel like it without regard for scheduling, and the pharmacy must stock the med cart on a regular basis.

What we are saying is: Don't allow your mental energy to be ruled by expectations. If you do, you can expect constant tension. Yes, hold people accountable. But don't feed a lot of energy into expecting people and things to be a certain way. That only sets you up for frustration and disappointment.

Be Process-Oriented

Another common cause of tension, and an energy robber, is being solely result-oriented rather than process-oriented. Of course, as nurses, we're trained to care about the results of our care and to put forth our best efforts; however, if all of our positive energy is suspended waiting for the task to be done, then we're missing the boat. *The Self-Health Guide: A Personal Program for Holistic Living* (Kripalu Publications, 1980, p. 112) expresses it this way:

> We often tend to focus so much of our energy and attention on the final result, that we do not and cannot enjoy the process. If we think all the time of how nice "it" will be when "it" is finished, or are anxious about the results, we take ourselves out of the present and lose the pleasure of the moment. Relaxation can only truly come when we are in the experience of the moment, not the thought of the future.

The irony is that all the anxiety we create over results can be avoided because the end result will naturally take care of itself if we are effective in the moment.

Maintain a Balance in Your Life

Let's look at the issue of how you use your energy. Have you ever found yourself saying things such as "It's not worth my energy to get annoyed," or "He's not worth getting upset over; my own health is more important," or "This task is not a good use of my energy, given all that needs to get done." At some level, we're plugged into the concept of how to spend our energy—and this becomes an imperative skill, given the energy the profession commands. The skill involved is wise choices at every turn. Nurses need to think of their energy as on a tight budget and be certain not to waste any of it. Why? Because you need every ounce you can get, not only to flow through the workday, but to have energy for your life, family, and friends beyond work. This brings up the whole issue of balance.

Maintaining balance in your life means *doing a healthy amount of the right thing.* Balance is about moderation. There needs to be a balance between work and play, sleep and wakefulness, time with others and time alone. Stop and think about what's out of balance in your life and beware of always having an excuse: "But I'm a student . . . but I'm a working mother . . . but I have a bad back." Kick those "buts" and do something to restore balance in your life because if you don't, this is what will happen: You will never replenish your energy pool, and your current energy supply will not only be low but will become stale and stagnated.

One additional comment about balance. *Balance* is a great word to use in keeping yourself in check throughout your workday. The word itself can bring you back to your center when you feel torn, troubled, or overwhelmed. Also remember that you can choose to remain centered and balanced even when others around you are not. Beware: Don't catch other people's stress!

Four Energy Traps

What else saps your energy? During the year prior to writing this book, we asked nurses this question, and they identified the following four energy traps as the most common: perfectionism, complaining, resisting reality, and judging.

The Perfectionism Trap

Many of your colleagues feel a real drive within to become the perfect nurse. But what does the perfect nurse look like, sound like, and act like? Are you trying to be that perfect nurse? Well, guess what? It's not working for your colleagues, and it's probably not working for you, either!

Once the parameters of perfectionism are defined, many nurses identify with the symptoms. Here's a quick quiz on some perfection items. Which ones are true for you?

	Yes	No
When you complete a project or task, do you remain satisfied only a short while before you want to start competing with yourself to change it or improve it?	☐	☐
Do you avoid new experiences (sports, hobbies) because you're afraid you won't be good enough?	☐	☐
Do you find yourself getting impatient and intolerant watching someone else tackle what you ordinarily do best?	☐	☐
Do you find failing painful and end up getting down on yourself?	☐	☐
Do you experience considerable guilt about not being the ideal nurse?	☐	☐
Do you hang on to standards that you measure yourself against when circumstances make such standards impossible to reach?	☐	☐
Do you have a gnawing feeling that whatever you do is never good enough?	☐	☐

How to interpret your responses: Add up all your yes responses. A total of seven yes responses is possible. If you have three or less, there's hope for you. You're growing roots of perfectionism, but you may be able to yank them out. Just be careful that they don't grow back!

If you have a score of four or more yes responses, you're perfectly hooked and have grown deep, strangulating roots of perfectionism. You're going to have to use some fairly drastic measures to be free of them.

We recommend that you turn over your soil completely, give up the need to be perfect, and watch the anxiety subside. The first step is to be conscious that perfectionism is an energy trap for you, and the second step is to *choose* not to fall into it.

Perfectionism can really be spelled P-A-R-A-L-Y-S-I-S. It traps our energy, and we end up immobilized in the present—afraid to try or unwilling to try because we're stuck on doing our work perfectly or want the perfect conditions. We also become immobilized by guilt—feeling bad, beating ourselves up because what we did wasn't good enough.

As a nurse, see if you can relate to any of the following examples of perfectionism:

Example 1	Yes	No
You withdraw or avoid patients' rooms sometimes because you don't have the perfect amount of time to give them the support and attention you think they need. So instead of doing something, you do nothing.	☐	☐

Example 2	Yes	No
You feel hurt by something a colleague said. You want to say the perfect thing to her or him. But you can't think of the words exactly, so you don't say anything.	☐	☐

Example 3	Yes	No
You have some ideas about solving a problem on the unit, but you hold back or give up improving the situation because it's not the *perfect* solution.	☐	☐

The key is to adopt some new mottoes—*"I'm perfectly imperfect"* and *"Don't wait to do your best—just DO!"*

The Complaining Trap

Another major energy waster is complaining. Are you a complainer? Maybe more than you care to admit? How about your unit? Is there a norm operating that says, "Let's all join together and complain"?

Complaining is a useless activity. We complain to others who can do nothing but endure our grumbling. In addition, it has a negative effect on the energy level of yourself and others. Have you ever noticed that we invest huge chunks of time complaining about things we have absolutely no control over, like the weather, the day's too long, it's only Monday, too many patients, too many call lights, and so forth?

So why do we complain? It seems like the thing to do. Maybe the best way to approach this question of "why" is to stop and answer it personally. Why do you complain? Check off the box near any statement in the following list that is true for you:

- ☐ Complaining is a means of getting acknowledgment for how hard I'm working.
- ☐ Complaining gets people to pay attention to me.
- ☐ Complaining justifies why I can't get more done.
- ☐ Complaining is a release for my frustration and tension.
- ☐ Complaining gets the higher-ups to take notice and to make necessary changes.
- ☐ Complaining helps me stay where I want to be, somewhat miserable.
- ☐ Complaining gives me something to talk about with people; otherwise, there would not be much to say.
- ☐ Complaining makes me feel better.
- ☐ Complaining substitutes nicely for getting involved in the sticky business of trying to change things or make things better.
- ☐ Complaining is a habit; I wouldn't know how to act differently.

Now look back over your check marks. Remember what we said before . . . we do things for reasons. You must be getting something from complaining; otherwise you wouldn't do it.

From an energy-conservation perspective, each time you engage in complaining, precious energy leaks out. Limiting or disabling thoughts consistently fed into the consciousness will produce the physical realities. In other words, what you expect is what you get. For example, "I'll never finish. It's impossible with all these interruptions," or "I have absolutely no pep today . . . I'll never survive the day. I'm tired before I begin." Do you hear it? Your mind is working against you, rather than for you.

In the list of 10 reasons you complain, there may be results attached to each reason that are valid and beneficial, that is, releasing frustration and tension, creating necessary change. The following are some antidotes to complaining that will allow you to get positive outcomes without the price of zapping your own energy and the energy of others:

- **Rationale: "Complaining is a release for my frustration and tension."**
  Antidote: Two-minute dump time. Pick a person to listen to you, someone who will simply serve as a sounding board and take two minutes in the beginning, middle, or end of your day and dump everything that you feel compelled to complain about. Imagine filling suitcases, each with a different set of problems. The idea is to dump the bags all at once instead of dragging them with you and having them contaminate your entire day and drain your energy bit by bit.
- **Rationale: "Complaining gets higher-ups to take notice and to make necessary changes."**
  Antidote: Request a meeting. Complaining may eventually serve your intent of getting those in charge to take note. However, a faster, more direct, and constructive approach would be to meet face-to-face with the people who have the power to change things. The meeting could simply serve the purpose of voicing frustrations and concerns. If you're in the dark about why things can't change, then your agenda would be to get an explanation.

The key is to *ask for what you need.* If you need someone to sound off to because you're sick and tired of being sick and tired, then ask. If you want to know the answers to troubling questions, then ask. It's always amazing how quick we are to say, "No one listens; no one tells me anything." And yet we never clearly asked for what we need. It's called taking the initiative. Don't stand passively by and point the finger.

Note: If you dismiss the antidote of requesting a meeting versus complaining, then consider this an important cue indicating one of the following: (1) The issue is a dead one. You need to bury it and move on. Or (2) you're not ready or willing to take action. Ask yourself if not, why not. Or (3) your complaints are, in truth, not as legitimate or as valid as you thought. Otherwise, you'd be willing to go public.

The Resisting Reality Trap

The third major trap that nurses reported as being a major energy robber is the resisting reality trap. See if you recognize the following signs of resisting reality. Do you ever find yourself upset, ruminating and festering about:

- What you don't like to do, but the reality is it's not going to go away, and there's no way around it.

Examples: doing paperwork, working holidays, being stuck in traffic.

- The way you expect the world to be, but it isn't.
Examples: there should be nurses out there to hire; patients should all be grateful; it's unfortunate that you can't walk the street at night and feel safe.
- The way you think things should go, but they don't.
Examples: supplies being on time; other nurses not calling in sick; large businesses providing child care arrangements for their employees.

We've all heard the saying, "Let go and go with the flow." This is what getting out of the resisting reality trap is all about—not fighting the "current" and not spending energy foolishly by being immobilized by things over which you have no control. All the resisting in the world is not going to change a thing.

Look over the following issues and see if any strikes a chord about an area in which you waste good energy by resisting reality:

	Yes	No
Resenting patients who push the call bell: Are call bells a reality?	☐	☐
Feeling angry about short staffing conditions: Is the nursing shortage a reality?	☐	☐
Being concerned about patients who take longer to care for because they're much sicker: Are sicker patients a reality?	☐	☐
Objecting to required attendance at in-service programs: Are in-service programs a reality?	☐	☐
Objecting to nursing positions that require working weekends and holidays: Is working weekends and holidays a reality for nurses?	☐	☐

We're not suggesting you shouldn't work at changing injustices, for change is at the heart of progress and growth. What we are asking is that you look at how much of your energy is wasted in allowing yourself to get stuck—spinning your wheels in frustration, anger, and procrastination about things that are out of your control. Even if you were to direct your best efforts, the chances of changing these conditions are slim.

The Point: Change the things you can. Let go of the things you can't. And have the wisdom to know the difference.

The Judging Mind Trap

Have you ever turned on a radio station that gradually seemed to get louder and louder and more offensive, until you finally found yourself abruptly turning it off and thinking to yourself (or, better yet, saying out loud), "Good grief! That's obnoxious!"

How does this radio station example relate to the judging mind? The fourth energy trap, the judging mind, can be like a constantly playing station in the background of our minds. Whatever or whoever comes into our field of awareness, the mind has the automatic tendency to pass judgment. For example, you meet someone for the first time. Your mind goes into full gear and instantly you produce a ticker tape of judgment: . . . She's pretty . . . she seemed bright . . . her teeth aren't great . . . nice smile . . . a little on the heavy side . . . great features . . . I didn't like her hairstyle . . . and so forth.

What are your spontaneous judgments about the people in your life? Think about them. What about your best friend? Your next door neighbor? A colleague you've known for a long time? Your manager? The head administrator? What characteristics do you automatically attribute to them the moment their name or face comes to mind?

What happened? Did you find your mind spinning out judgments left and right? It's rather astounding when you come to realize the magnitude of this phenomenon.

The judging mind is our inner dialogue. It compliments, criticizes, evaluates, accepts, or rejects anything and everyone that comes into our field of awareness.

There are two major negative effects of the judging mind:

1. **The judging mind contributes greatly to fatigue and exhaustion.** The mind needs a break. Some days we have the judging-mind station turned up so loud that it's like a kid gone crazy in the penny arcade, feeding one quarter after the next for hours upon hours—morning until night.

2. **The judging mind is the gateway for the manifestation of our reality.** Your mind is a combination judge, jury, and executioner. If you have, for example, heavy negative judgments about some doctor, it's fairly predictable that those judgments will determine the success or failure of that working relationship. Think about it: Every time the guy walks onto the unit, your mind starts blasting off the judgment: "Here comes that jerk . . . he's a true idiot . . . he thinks he's so cool . . . he probably wears his stethoscope to bed at night." Now ask yourself, is your relationship with that doctor going to be wonderful?

In essence, the judging mind draws us closer to people or pulls us away. The judging mind opens our hearts and minds to communicate and trust, or it shuts the mind and heart down and dis-engages. As you can see, we're not talking about just a small energy trap here. The judging mind has far-reaching and powerful implications.

The response, then, is to adopt a state of neutrality, as discussed in chapter 5, "Stress: A Critical Course." *Neutrality* is simply a concept of a mind that has been retrained not to judge one way or the other. The mind simply pushes the neutral button and does not enter into judgment, period. It's a mind discipline—a mind control. Neutrality, we believe, is a skill that needs to be practiced and integrated gradually as a way of being and a way of thinking.

The practice of neutrality, at the very least, will save you substantial energy. At best, it can open the door to a world of greater vitality, fulfillment, and joy.

Summary

The purpose of this chapter has been to give you an opportunity to take stock of where you might be trapping, losing, or wasting energy and to assist you in reestablishing your role as the person responsible for how you use your energy. We want to encourage you to exercise conscious responses, not only with regard to how you spend energy but also with regard to how you conserve your energy.

Insight and awareness of these potential energy traps is half the battle. The other half is won by being truly committed to sustaining positive energy. That requires exercising thoughts, feelings, and actions that are energy boosters rather than energy traps. Energy traps not only incapacitate our minds but also drag down the body and dampen the spirit of life. That state of having a low level of energy makes us unhappy and unhealthy, not to mention inefficient.

Why not create a new campaign for yourself that compels you to climb out of the energy traps, once and for all, and jump on a bandwagon of energy boosters! It's up to you, and the time is now!

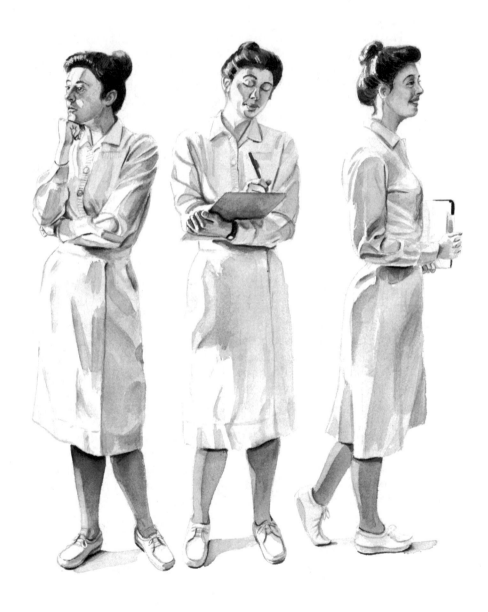

Chapter 7

The How-to's of Working Smarter

Has the thought ever crossed your mind that work is too time- and energy-consuming to just "endure" it? So many nurses are searching for ways to make work more satisfying and less frustrating. After all, you probably entered the nursing profession with expectations of gratification and fulfillment.

What happened? Certainly the external environment has changed. But that's only one source of disillusionment. In today's complex society, many of us have lost touch with the knowledge of how to use our abilities to lead satisfying and meaningful work lives.

This chapter focuses on you and the power of your own inner nature to nurture peaceful, productive, and satisfying work habits.

What Motivates You?

To understand the philosophy that underlies working smarter, it helps to consider your motivation behind your work. What motivates you? Your first response may be your paycheck . . . naturally. The paycheck is an *external* motivator. What else motivates you? Your desire to help others? Altruism is an *internal* motivator. Consider the differences between external and internal motivators and their effects on your job satisfaction and happiness.

On the whole, we live in a society that emphasizes the external motivators such as the trappings of success, career ladders, status, prestige, power, and financial compensation. We live in a world that moves exceedingly fast. And while some of us prefer not to live this way, we get caught up in the fast lane, and escape seems almost impossible.

We value our freedom; yet inside we may be prisoners of tension and pressure. We end up paying a high price for this way of life by growing out of touch with ourselves, our own pace, and our natural gifts and abilities. We move so fast that we don't take time to appreciate ourselves. We end up defining and measuring our success in life by what we do, instead of valuing who we are.

Our need for status and accomplishment often expresses an overriding need for acceptance or approval. If we're motivated by the need for acceptance and approval, we live in fear of not getting enough. It's hard to bring our motives to conscious awareness, because these patterns are ingrained very early in life. Remember when you felt good about yourself if you got an A and bad about yourself if you got a C or a D?

Many nurses acknowledge in themselves a preoccupation with whether they're "getting their due" in terms of status, pay, and recognition. Given the flux in the nursing profession, it's not easy to be free of this defensive posture. Yet, this stance depletes most nurses' feelings of significance. The volume is turned up so loud on these external motivators that we have literally drowned out the internal motivators that contribute to job gratification and sense of purpose.

What are *your* internal motivators? What makes you tick from the inside out? What compels you to do all you can as a nurse? Is it your desire to help others? To use your gifts and talents? To express your love and joy? To experience personal growth and expansion? To be responsible in your life? You probably can add more of your own internal motivators to this list.

If you are feeling empty, restless, or disillusioned as a nurse, consider turning your attention from external to internal motivators. As Tarthang Tulku (*Skillful Means*, Dharma Publishing, Berkeley, California, 1978, p. 4) so aptly puts it:

> By focusing our energy outside of ourselves, we miss the many internal messages from our senses, from our thoughts, feelings, and perceptions. Without this inner knowledge and the freedom it provides, our attitude towards our experience grows shallow, and our awareness loses depth and clarity.
>
> Even though we may be successful in the world, a separation from our real nature leaves us without a sound internal foundation on which we can base our lives. This leads us to subtle feelings of insecurity, and life can begin to seem empty and meaningless.

How can you get back in tune with yourself and experience deeper satisfaction and happiness from work? Practice the four how-to's of working smarter, and you'll gradually discover a wellspring of satisfaction and happiness you might have forgotten was there. If you're expecting a typical bombardment of time-management techniques, you're wrong. This material is about a different kind of smarts.

Four Skills for Working Smarter

These four skills are:

- Inner observation
- Mindfulness
- Going directly into your work
- Embracing all of your work

Skill 1: Inner Observation

Inner observation involves awareness of each thought and feeling that accompanies whatever you're doing at every given moment. Think of it as watching the activity of your mind and heart. You become an observer of your own inner nature. When you observe your inner nature thoughtfully, you experience a release of tension and, in turn, bring about a sense of calmness, ease, and relaxation. It's like a gentle energy flow.

Try it right now. Tune in to what you're thinking and feeling as you read this book. Don't stop whatever you're doing. Just be aware of what you're thinking and feeling as you go along. You'll feel centered or balanced as you go about your business.

Begin to tune in to your tasks and responsibilities at work with regard to how you're helping others. As you do something routine, bring your full consciousness to it. For example, if you are helping a patient with a bath, savor in your thoughts, feelings, and actions how much better the patient will feel when he or she is clean and refreshed.

Or, if you're writing a memo, contemplate as you're doing it how well-informed and helped the recipient is going to feel, even if she does not respond. As Tarthang Tulku suggests in *Skillful Means* (p. 8):

> The strength and awareness we gain in this way gives us control over the direction and purpose of our lives. All of our actions reflect a natural cheerfulness, and life and work take on a light,

enjoyable quality that sustains us in everything we do. Life becomes an art, an expression of the flowing interactions of our bodies, mind, and senses with each experience in our lives. We can rely on ourselves to fulfill even our innermost needs and, thus, we become genuinely free. Inner freedom allows us to use our intelligence wisely; once we learn how to use it, we can never lose the clarity and confidence it brings.

Skill 2: Mindfulness

Mindfulness involves concentrating on *one task at a time* and centering all of your attention on what you are doing in every detail.

Mindfulness is a combination of:

- Concentration
- Clarity
- Awareness

This concentration should not be imposed with strict discipline. Rather, it should be done with lightness and ease. When distractions enter your mind, just gently let them pass through. Let them go.

Mindfulness also means your energy is focused. When you learn to focus energy and work at the gut level, each minute is an important part of the task, and you learn to measure time carefully. The principle here is "to be in the moment." If you're not in the "now," you rob the present by being caught up in yesterday or worrying about tomorrow. Getting in touch with your "now" is at the heart of effective work. When you think about it, there is literally no other moment you can live fully.

As Wayne Dyer suggests in *Your Erroneous Zones* (Avon Books, New York City, 1977, p. 24):

> The present moment, that elusive time which is always with you, can be the most beautifully experienced if you allow yourselves to get lost in it. Drink in all of every moment and tune out that past which is over and the future which will arrive in time.

When you're "in the moment," time itself seems to expand. You are able to work more efficiently, and yet speech loses its rushed and frantic quality. Through concentration and mindfulness, you become better organized and use each available moment to its maximum. When you succeed in experiencing the rhythm of mindfulness, you quickly recognize lapses or slips and the effects these have on the quality of your work experience.

Mindfulness has many benefits. It brings grace to your movements, organization to your thoughts, and satisfying results to your efforts. Mindfulness involves shifting from a scattered mind to a focused mind, bringing concentrated attention to each task and completing it before starting the next.

Concentration sounds easy, but it's not. It takes mental discipline and retraining the mind to focus and be on purpose. The mind has a tendency to wander. It's like a helium balloon—if you don't hold on to the string of your mind, it floats and drifts, dispersing and fragmenting your mental energy, instead of focusing it on your work.

Have you ever had the experience of performing a task, but then, within a few short minutes, not being able to recall doing it at all. Your body went through the motions, but your mind scattered in many directions. At the patient's bedside, do you ever go through the motions of a procedure and yet fail to connect with the patient? It's as if the patient were not there, because *you* were somewhere else!

The less focused you are, the less satisfaction you reap, and lack of concentration is reflected in the quality of your results. Do you recognize any of these symptoms in your work when you are not being mindful? For example:

- ☐ It takes longer to get things done.
- ☐ I make more mistakes.
- ☐ I forget and lose things.
- ☐ I jump from one task to another, leaving things unfinished.
- ☐ I feel overwhelmed and out of control.
- ☐ I allow myself to get sidetracked and distracted.
- ☐ I end up distracting others.
- ☐ I waste time.

How to Develop Mindfulness

The following is some advice on how to develop mindfulness:

- **When you begin work, take a moment or two to breathe in gently and slowly.** Be aware of your breath as it enters and leaves your body. As you inhale, think of it as grounding your energy and calming your mind.
- **Consider your priorities and assume they will shift throughout the day.** Don't fight it. Anticipate it and flow with it.

- **Take things one at a time.**
- **Ignore distractions by becoming absorbed with each detail of your work as you're doing it.** When irrelevant thoughts interrupt, think of them as clouds, letting them drift out.
- **When your mind wanders, gently bring it back to the task before you.**
- **Take joy in the task at hand; don't postpone appreciation to the end.** Real satisfaction is there . . . in the process. By focusing only on results, you often end up disappointed. Meanwhile, you miss the joy in the present moment.

Skill 3: Going Directly into Your Work

Going directly into your work means not holding back, hesitating, putting off, avoiding, or procrastinating. So often, nurses are faced with a difficult or busy day. You react by imposing limits about what you can get done. Anxiety sets in and obstructs your efforts. As Tarthang Tulku states in *Skillful Means* (p. 20):

> When we grow nervous and tense, our perceptions become clouded so we can no longer see clearly what needs to be done. We become scattered and inefficient, which, in turn, makes us tired and tense. Anxiety and tension take the place of significant action and simply drain our energy away. We find ourselves worried about our work rather than dealing with it directly. Our worrying takes so much of our energy that we can no longer respond openly to the demands of each new situation. Our minds constrict our bodies in patterns of physical tension, which make it even more difficult to work effectively or with enjoyment. As anxiety replaces pleasure of work, we find we have little space to find enjoyment in our lives and little to give to others.

Do You Hold Back?

Think about your work day and ways that you hold back. Maybe it's a demanding patient whom you greet halfheartedly, or a colleague whom you could compliment but don't. Or perhaps you put off things that need to be done, such as charting at the time you deliver care, or ordering that piece of lamb's wool to alleviate a patient's bedsore. Do you avoid tasks you don't like to do, such as getting a stool specimen or calling maintenance to come and fix a patient's overhead light? What kind of things do *you* procrastinate about? Signing up for that mandatory in-service? Completing that special assignment? Calling in the family members for a much-needed conference?

If any of these examples ring true for you, consider the energy you're wasting. Can you see how your work rhythm becomes interrupted and disturbed? Just by making the choice not to hold back but to go directly into your work, you expand your energy. Even when you're tired, by plunging into all the work at hand and not avoiding it, you find renewed vitality because you're using your energy consistently.

By bringing your full energy of mind and heart to your work, you become involved deeply. When you hold back or bring only half-hearted energy to what you do, you drift or stay on the surface, never going deeply enough into your work to find true gratification. In *Skillful Means* (p. 18), Tarthang Tulku states:

> A routine task done with all your energy will be more satisfying than a half-hearted involvement in a more demanding project. You will discover that what makes the difference in your work is the attitude with which you do it. As you become more effective in doing simple things well, you can improve your ability to plan and set wise goals, and you can carry out more complex goals with ease.

Skill 4: Embracing All of Your Work

Embracing all of your work means not placing a higher value on some tasks than on others, not discriminating between what is easier/harder, more important/less important, more prestigious/less prestigious. Embracing all of your work means encompassing it all and going directly from one responsibility to the next without engaging in all the mental gymnastics in between.

You might think that you're better off avoiding hard work and saving your energy for the things you like to do. This is a fallacy, because success and satisfaction come from *effort*. By picking and choosing, by accepting and rejecting, by starting and stopping, you end up wasting your energy and interrupting the rhythm and tone of your work.

If you learn to embrace all of your work, you encourage rather than defeat yourself. When your mind cranks out thoughts such as "I hate doing that," or "That's a bore," or "Any idiot could do this job," simply decide to call a halt to that way of thinking. Cancel these thoughts as if they never occurred, and move on. As Tarthang Tulku suggests in *Skillful Means* (p. 31):

Instead of looking at our work as an enemy to be conquered, we can embrace the many challenges it affords us. When we do this, we can focus our energy in a light and pleasurable way, and it's much easier to persist in a task until we have reached our goal. When we work in this way, we learn to appreciate even work we dislike doing.

Now What? The Challenge

The challenge now is to integrate the skills of working smarter into your work life. At some level, you're already experiencing these steps and have already tasted the benefits. Now you simply need to bring heightened consciousness of how to work smarter into your every-day work.

Practice the how-to's of working smarter out of your desire to grow rather than out of a need to "repair your deficiencies." In *Mrs. Warren's Profession*, George Bernard Shaw expressed it this way:

> People are always blaming their circumstances for what they are. I don't believe in circumstances. The people who get on in this world are the people who get up and look for the circumstances they want, and if they can't find them, make them.

The skills of working smarter involve changing your consciousness at work. It's possible, but it takes practice, practice, practice . . . and more patience. Just as you can't learn to run a four-minute mile overnight, you can't train yourself to engage in new mental behavior immediately after you read about it and theoretically understand it. Instead, you need to unlearn the old and relearn the new way of thinking. In order to do this, you need to commit yourself to your own happiness and repeat endlessly that your mind is your own and you are capable of training it to work smarter.

Then, train yourself in one skill at a time for working smarter. For instance, print one skill on a three-by-five-inch index card and carry it in your uniform pocket, changing the skill each week. Post the card on your mirror, tape it on your dashboard, place it under a magnet on your refrigerator. Bombard yourself with reminders. Begin to apply the four skills of working smarter, and you'll experience immediate results. Keep developing the skills by reviewing this chapter periodically to imprint these powerful concepts into your mind.

Summary

This chapter has been about how to achieve a more satisfying, more productive professional life by becoming a more internally motivated person. We have demonstrated that deeper satisfaction and happiness as a nurse come from being "centered" and choosing to participate 100 percent in your life and in your work. Remember, the deeper the involvement, the greater the professional satisfaction.

We have introduced the four skills for working smarter, including the concept of mindfulness as a way of focusing your energy to "be in the moment" and to go directly into your work, avoiding the prime energy waster of procrastination.

Practice the four skills for working smarter, and you'll steadily experience a calmer, more peaceful, and more productive self. You're going to feel good about the way you're getting the job done! Remember—it's all in the practice. So, let's go for it!

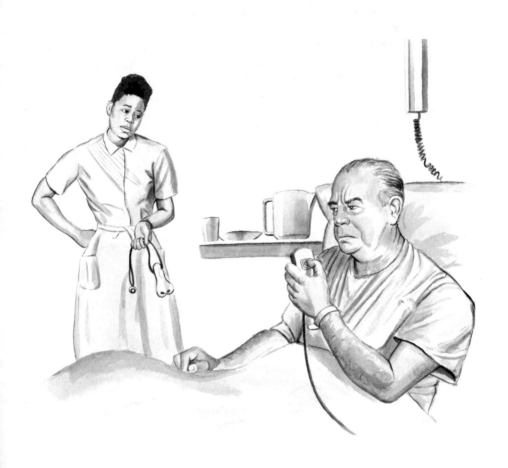

Chapter 8

The Patient as Customer

A potentially damaging clash of values is occurring between patients and health care organizations. This clash involves everyone working in health care, particularly nurses. Nurses report feeling a great deal of resistance to giving patients *service* as opposed to nursing *care*. The roots of this clash between patients and nurses lie in our historical tradition of altruism and advocacy and in our emerging professionalism and our new need to respond to the patient as a customer. In this chapter, the historical roots of resistance to the concept of service are explored in an effort to help incorporate service into professional practice.

To understand this clash of values, let's step back and look at the broader picture of the health care market today. Think about the structure of your facility—its organizational chart. Who is at the top? And who is at the bottom?

You probably answered that the board of directors or the chief executive officer is at the top and the patient is at the bottom. In your interactions with patients and their families recently, would you say that they see themselves at the bottom of the organization? Definitely not!

But if you attend directors' or administrators' meetings, you seldom hear the word "patient" mentioned. In fact, one administrator, Travis Cross of Portland, Oregon, made a sign that said "B.W.A.T.P.?" and put it on the table during meetings to remind himself and others about their purpose. The sign stands for "But What About The Patient?"

Nurses are not exempt from forgetting about the patient, either. Postgraduation idealism wears off, and reality shock sets in. It seems impossible to be the professional nurse you expected to be and to give patients the care you were taught to give in school. The demands on your time often seem to conflict with your purpose. Chances are that you have been on contact overload a thousand times. It's very easy to become jaded.

We've asked nurses all over the country to demonstrate the realities of their work, and this is what we were told over and over again: The patient often gets the least attention as nurses spin from one *immediate* demand or task to another. Nurses express anger, frustration, confusion, and sadness about this state of affairs. It is sad . . . and it doesn't have to be that way.

Patients intend to make sure they don't continue to be treated as though they're on the bottom of the organizational chart. A new customer mind-set among patients is part of the sweeping changes affecting health care. Patients have a different attitude about health care, and this includes a different attitude toward doctors and nurses. Patients also have expectations of their care, which they sometimes express adamantly. This new posture evokes feelings in nurses that conflict with traditional values of altruism about the patient and the patient-advocate role of the nurse.

What is your vision for nursing? Do you think that we are better off as a result of the massive changes happening in health care? How do you feel about the new attitude of patients?

What is vision, anyway? Vision is your picture of the future and what you hope for. The future could be the next hour, the next week, or the next 50 years. Vision gives you direction. It shapes your values and guides your actions.

"Whether our vision of nursing is one of science, caring, or some mixture of both, it always includes nurses and patients." This quote is from Karen Buhler-Wilkerson and Julie Fairman, in the article "Missing data: nurses with their patients" [*Nursing Research* 36(1):38, January–February 1987]. The basis of the profession is its commitment to caring. Nurses repeatedly identify the patient as a primary source of reward. In the midst of burgeoning social, political, and professional change, this book supports the nurse in exploring the impact of these changes on the nurse-patient relationship. Our approach stems from a tradition of caring and attempts to help move the profession forward through a time of painful transition.

Where Did the Patients Go?

In preliminary research, we asked 200 nurses if their patients today differ from those of five years ago. Ninety-five percent said yes emphatically. Most nurses stated that although the patient is a major source of personal and professional reward, some changes in their patients are a source of conflict.

How have patients changed? They are:

- Sicker
- More questioning
- Less trusting
- More knowledgeable
- Demanding of good service and care
- Willing to shop around
- Discharged sooner
- Older
- More cost-conscious
- More demanding
- Quicker to sue

In short, many of your contemporaries agreed that the patient today is acting more like a *customer*. This change represents a significant shift in the patient's power. Patients no longer see themselves as passive, dependent recipients of care. They have rising expectations of their health care and of nurses.

Do you think this change in the patient—this rising customer consciousness—is a fad? In our experience, we have found that nurses do not see it as a fad and, in fact, think the shift in power is only just beginning to affect the health care system and the nursing profession. It seems critically important to us that we understand and move beyond a resistance to service as a part of professional practice.

A Welcome Change?

What is *your* reaction to treating the patient as a consumer or customer? And why is there this resistance to treating the patient as a customer? Five trends in nursing shed light on this:

- **Trend 1: From Handmaiden to Practitioner**
- **Trend 2: From Volunteer to Professional**
- **Trend 3: From High-Touch to High-Tech**
- **Trend 4: From Authority to Facilitator**
- **Trend 5: From a Clinical Service to a Business**

Trend 1: From Handmaiden to Practitioner

Nursing has moved from a position of dependence upon the physician for complete direction to one of growing independent nursing practice. Nurses no longer stand up when a physician enters the room. We no longer rely solely on *medical research* to direct clinical practice. Nurses now make judgments on the basis of nursing research and our training as nurses. We are defining our own areas of nursing practice. Primary nursing represents an effort to publicly assume responsibility for nursing care and to be accountable for the outcomes of nursing actions. The idea of providing a service to patients may be perceived as demeaning in the face of this new emerging status as an independent practitioner.

Trend 2: From Volunteer to Professional

It used to be that women volunteered their time to care for the sick. Nursing was either a female pastime to be set aside for marriage and child rearing, or a suitable occupation during periods of war. Rapid technological advances in medicine and health care emphasized the need for further, formal nursing education. Now, education in hospital-based schools of nursing is giving way to associate- and baccalaureate-degree programs. Emulating the other professions of law and medicine, the nursing profession has established standards of clinical practice and licensure requirements. The behaviors of nurses are increasingly governed by law and by professional organizations. The trend is toward increasing self-governance and autonomy.

Service, on the other hand, is often associated with nonprofessional occupations requiring little or no formal education. At a time when nurses are asserting a right to higher status and pay commensurate with high levels of responsibility, service behaviors and attitudes may seem regressive.

Trend 3: From High-Touch to High-Tech

Without technical knowledge to guide practice, nurses once relied primarily on touch, intuition, and nurturing to care for patients. Today, nursing is done on the basis of technological skill and scientific knowledge. Incident reports are filed on errors of omission or errors in technical skill or practice, not for omissions of empathy, delays in answering call lights, or lack of respect and humaneness. This trend mirrors our society, which traditionally has deemphasized "feminine" skills in favor of more "masculine" technological skills. Service, then, is often linked with devalued worth, both of the work and of the person who performs it.

Since the profession has gained stature by the acquisition of scientific knowledge and technological skills, the services patients seem to be demanding (empathy, hot tea, flower vases, and the like) feel like a regression to the handmaiden stage or a reversal to the days of nurturing, not technological skill. These demands are also occurring at a time when nursing's resources to deliver excellent care are shrinking, and all demands are on the rise.

Trend 4: From Authority to Facilitator

Many authors have written about the patient's historically dependent position within the health care system. Not many writers focus on the authority of nurses over patients and our ambivalence at losing this position of power and control. The role of the nurse is moving away from control toward that of facilitator.

Patients became "clients," a term that publicly recognized their right to participate in planning care. Nurses began to work more collaboratively with patients and their families. Change in the patient's power didn't seem problematic until empowered patients began to challenge nursing's control and to act like consumers. Patients now demand a response. The nurse no longer gives from a position of benevolence or collaboration; she or he is compelled to respond. This expectation of response can clash with the nurse's emerging identity as a skilled, knowledgeable professional.

Just as the profession is rising in stature, the patient steals the show and grabs the power. In our new role as independent, accountable practitioners, it is natural to want to "strut our stuff," to want patients to recognize our skills and contributions. Some nurses believe that it would be detrimental to the profession to respond positively to patient demands for skilled care and amenities. They believe that it would weaken our hard-won power and authority.

Trend 5: From a Clinical Service to a Business

The clinical service that nurses provided to patients used to be organized around delivering prescribed care to patients. Each unit had a head nurse who knew all of the patients and closely scrutinized their care. This head nurse also knew all of the staff well. The same physicians admitted patients to the unit and knew the nurses by name. Depending on the size of the unit and the way care was organized, the head nurse or the team leaders or both would make rounds with the physicians. Physicians knew who to talk to about their patients' care.

This picture hardly exists today. Health care has become a big business concerned with profits, efficiency, productivity, cost containment, quality, and competitive position in the industry. The head nurse has acquired the new title of "manager" and with it new 24-hour accountability and responsibility for the budget and quality assurance. The manager of today might have as many as 60 employees and responsibility for a six-figure budget containing personnel and nonpersonnel line items, attend an equal number of meetings as nonnursing personnel, and continue to be responsible for the care given by nurses.

Staff nurses are also asked to seek more efficient, cost-effective ways to deliver care to patients. Productivity and cost containment are critical issues in evaluating a unit's performance.

Nurses, although supportive of the patient's acquisition of power and legitimate right to demand service, fear an inability to be responsive to both the patient and the institution for whom they work. Because of the dramatic changes brought about by prospective payment, patients are sicker, fewer nursing positions are budgeted (a fact only compounded by the latest nursing shortage), support services have fewer employees to deliver supplies, and supplies are scarce. The demands by the institution for nurses to wear more hats and perform more nonnursing functions are increasing. A common cry from nurses in response to the above is, "I can't do it all. There isn't enough time for service, too!"

Resistance Beliefs

The consumer movement in health care is a fact, not a fad. Nurses need to find a way to move forward and respond to the expectations of their customers. Each nurse has much to gain from coming to terms with resistance toward giving excellent "service" as part and parcel of excellent, professional nursing care.

Here are four commonly held "resistance beliefs" that we have heard repeatedly from nurses on the topic of service excellence:

- The focus on service will make airline attendants or waitresses out of nurses.
- The focus on service degrades the profession in the eyes of other health care workers, especially physicians.
- The emphasis on service gives patients permission to be more demanding and make even more unreasonable requests of nurses.
- The pressure to give service to patients takes more time and staff.

As a professional, you need to think through these beliefs about giving excellent service to patients and decide where you stand. Just as you have choices about your thoughts and feelings, you have options regarding whether you adopt or reject these resistance beliefs:

- **Belief 1: Giving service and meeting the patient's needs makes waitresses or airline attendants out of nurses who consider themselves to be professionals.** From our work with nursing groups, we have learned that, by and large, nurses believe nursing needs to take responsibility for the profession's image among its own members first. You possess intellectual, interpersonal, and communication skills that distinguish your activities from other service providers. Remember the quote by Eleanor Roosevelt, "No one can make you feel inferior without your consent." Care of patients has always involved service, and still the profession has grown in stature. Openly stating that service is a part of professional practice doesn't change the nature of the job; it is only one part of your work. If you have a professional image of yourself that includes your service role, the public will see it and respect it.

At the outset of the health care service excellence movement, proponents equated hospitals with hotels, regarding patients as "guests," and attempted to provide a service atmosphere of courtesy and convenience analogous to that of the hotel industry. Nurses who tried to conform to this analogy, however, understood that it falls short in several key ways. The nature of the health care consumer is different, as are the circumstances of the visit and the expected outcomes (figure 8-1). The current concept of service excellence as a

Figure 8-1. Differences between Customers in Hotels and Hospitals

In Hotels	In Hospitals
Most people are there voluntarily.	Health considerations force admission.
Most people are in a good mood.	Most patients feel irritable, exposed, anxious, and scared.
Many people are on expense accounts.	Many patients are panicked about the high costs.
Guests expect pampering and convenience.	Customers expect complex technological know-how to save life, and also expect compassion.
Employees must be courteous and responsive.	Employees must be safe, accurate, skilled, careful, compassionate, kind, alert, quick, responsive, and much more.

Source: Reprinted, with permission, from Leebov, W. *Service Excellence: The Customer Relations Strategy for Health Care,* published by American Hospital Publishing, Inc., copyright 1988, p. 27.

customer relations approach to health care respects these differences between patient and hotel guest, while respecting the patient's role as a discriminating consumer.

In view of the emerging importance of service excellence and of patients as customers, a comprehensive plan of care includes an assessment of the physiological and emotional health factors of the patient, the nursing actions required to restore the patient to a state of optimum health, and an individualized care plan. If service were the only thing you did as a nurse, the public might see you as a waitress, but service is just one component of a comprehensive plan of care, and it is a component that contributes to the patient's well-being—it is that extra cup of coffee you give to a nervous patient or the empathy you provide to a worried patient.

- **Belief 2: Giving service further degrades the nursing profession in the eyes of other professionals, especially doctors.** Nursing groups report that this belief is invalid because all health care professionals, including physicians, are more conscious of service, and it is important to remaining competitive in today's market. No one in health care, especially nurses, is immune to the need to treat patients as customers. The reality of today's market requires strong relationships with patients. As consumers, patients have the power to choose other health care providers if you don't satisfy them.

- **Belief 3: Service emphasis gives patients permission to be even more demanding.** A positive attitude toward patients' persistent requests enables you to look more deeply at their need to call out (sometimes yell) for help. Don't stop at the surface of this behavior. It's probably a red flag signaling a deeper issue.

    Patients' demands often disguise a need for support. Part of their need to demand might originate in our failure to meet previous needs. Alternatively, perhaps their expectation that we'll fail them is made on the basis of their experience during a previous admission or what they learned from friends. It might also stem from blatant fear. People cope differently with their feelings associated with illness and hospitalization. For some, being demanding is one way to incite people to take care of them.

    Failure to meet patients' demands compounds their lack of trust. On the other hand, responding fully to the patient deepens their trust in you and allows you to fully appreciate your own skills.

- **Belief 4: The service emphasis will take more time and staff.** This is a hard belief to counter because of the severity of the nursing shortage. This belief may be valid. However, there are ways to give excellent service to patients even within limits. For example, you can be mentally and emotionally present with the patient no matter how long the interaction lasts. You can make excellent the service you have control over and let go of the frustration associated with attempting to control areas of service you cannot control. Ask yourself honestly how much extra service you could give to patients if you fully embraced all of your work.

  Make the most of your work. Take time in the short run to make time in the long run. Research has shown that patients are more cooperative when nurses convey warmth, courtesy, and personal treatment. These behaviors reduce patient anxiety and provide a supportive climate for healing and recovery. An insecure, anxious patient in the long run is more demanding, harder to please, and more time-consuming.

Patient Demands: An Opportunity in Disguise?

Even though higher salaries and recognition for nurses are long overdue, not all nurses are pessimistic about what's happening in nursing today. Nurse managers may be disappointed with the amount of time spent on staffing issues, but they are enthusiastic about their autonomy and new roles. Many nurses are turning patients' demands for service into opportunities for greater personal reward.

For example, Janet, a nurse we spoke with, described coming on duty at 7:30 one morning and listening to the night staff complain in report about a particular patient's wife. "Mrs. Garrity was upset," one night nurse was griping, "because I couldn't bring her a cup of tea. I was in the middle of trying to restart two IVs!"

Before report was over, the same patient's light was on. This time, Mr. Garrity's daughter had brought flowers and wanted a vase. Janet got the vase and spent five minutes thanking the daughter and Mrs. Garrity for the care and attention they gave to the patient. Mrs. Garrity began to berate the night nurse for having a bad attitude. Janet listened without attempting to justify the other nurse's bahavior. Then she told Mrs. Garrity she would follow up with the night nurse and asked if they or Mr. Garrity needed anything more at the moment. She repeated her appreciation for their attention to the patient.

It was at that point that Janet learned the patient had grown the roses the daughter had brought in and that gardening was his favorite pastime.

When Mr. Garrity died, his wife made a special effort to write to Janet to tell her how meaningful Janet had been to the family during her husband's last days in the hospital. The letter balanced some of the feelings of guilt Janet had experienced because she couldn't spend extended periods of time with this patient. It was just this kind of incident that Janet would draw on in difficult times to remind her how much gratification she derived from her role as a nurse.

Exercise 1

Reconsider your ideas about each of the four resistance beliefs. Identify concrete behaviors that will answer patients' needs and increase your rewards from your work. For example, design a personal strategy for dealing with patients who are difficult for you to care for. Present this to your nurse manager and coworkers to adopt as a unit standard of care. Brainstorm about ways to approach difficult patients that might reduce or change their negative behavior. Use your creative imagination to transform a problem into an opportunity. Here are examples to help get you started:

- **Make the most of the moment.** Use the giving of medication as an opportunity to touch patients, smile, or ask a question about their care.
- **Do what you need to do in a personal, attentive way.** While you change an IV, for example, notice something about the patient that you can discuss.
- **Take action on your options.** If the supplies are not there when you need them, inform your nurse manager and perform some other part of the patient's care.

Exercise 2

Think of a patient you cared for in the past three months, someone who was difficult to work with. Use this exercise to set the stage for your next encounter with a similar patient. This exercise works even better when you have just had your first difficult interaction. Ask yourself these questions:

1. What creates the feeling of difficulty?
2. What opportunity for growth does the behavior offer you?
3. Have you looked at the situation deeply enough? How complete is your understanding of the patient? What thoughts about the patient can you change?

4. Identify your options. What new actions can you take to turn the next incident into an opportunity for responsibility, appreciation, and a deeper understanding of yourself?

As discussed in chapter 1, "Taking Charge," change is a difficult process that requires commitment. Commit yourself to the new actions and options you've indicated above.

Your work offers an opportunity to learn more about yourself and incorporate higher values into your daily experience. By caring for your work and responding to it fully, you exercise your talents and abilities and contribute your energy to life. Responding to the patients' needs is a professional action that also helps you advance toward personal goals.

Emerson said that what lies behind you and what lies before you pale in significance when compared to what lies within you. This is even more true when you take responsibility for your response to life's situations. Instead of blaming the patient for thinking like a customer, let's feel gratitude toward the patient for the opportunity to grow and appreciate our work as professionals.

In a 1987 editorial commemorating the 35th anniversary issue of *Nursing Research*, Florence Downs calls upon nurses to make a "reaffirmation of our commitment to caring." The integration of service excellence and professional practice is a step toward that commitment. Commit yourself to excellence in those areas of practice you control. The personal and professional rewards are endless.

Summary

This chapter has discussed the resistance of nurses to the growing emphasis on customer service in the health care industry. We have made suggestions on how a customer service orientation can be made compatible with the growing sense of professionalism among nurses.

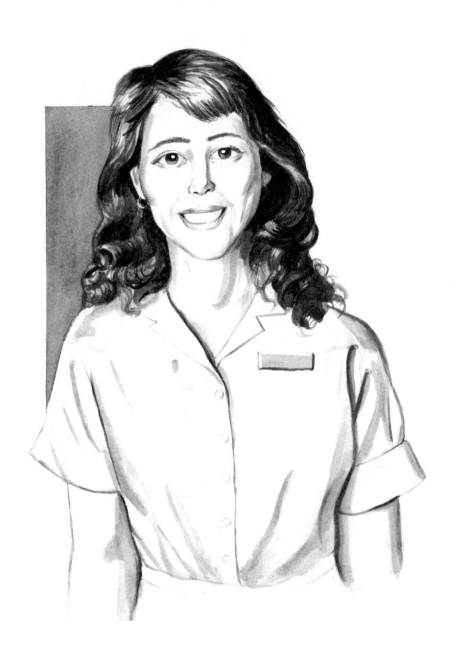

Chapter 9

Change

This brings us to the last chapter in the book. We hope that you have gained new insights into yourself and reconfirmed previous ideas. Perhaps your journey through the book has helped you to identify new ways to get what you want in your life and in your work. For some people, the challenge of change is exciting. For others, perhaps most of us, it is linked with feelings of dread and anxiety.

All of us have tried to change something about ourselves and have discovered that our attempts to be different have failed. (How many diets have you been on?) Why are some of your attempts to change successful and others futile? Before you set off on another attempt, let's look at two prerequisites for change that may help you to be more successful this time.

Do you know anyone who is perfect? You probably know a lot of people who are unhappy with themselves for not being "just right." You may be one of them. It is very hard to change if you don't like yourself. Self-acceptance is the first prerequisite for lasting change.

Self-acceptance and being perfect are not the same things. You may still want to become better at something, or you may want to reduce or eliminate a thought or behavior you have. But, at the same time, self-acceptance is appreciating yourself for *everything* you are right now, saying, "This is all of me, and I like myself for who I am."

Everyone has parts of their personality, including their behavior, that they would like to strengthen. It is much easier to do that with a positive attitude than with a negative one. As we described earlier, negative thoughts, especially disabling self-thoughts, lead to the Self-

Defeating Zone. Positive change is very difficult to initiate from that place.

If you find that you are intolerant of parts of yourself, spend your initial energy working to achieve a position of neutrality and then acceptance of every part of you. It would help if you spent time thinking about what you gain from thinking negatively about yourself. That statement may sound odd, but people who do something usually have a reason. People think and act to get what they need; when you are honest with yourself about what you get from thinking negatively about some part of yourself, you can make a conscious choice about whether you want it and, if so, what else you could do to get it.

Once you have accepted all of yourself, you are ready for the second prerequisite to change: a deep desire to change. If you look back at your last unsuccessful attempt to change something, ask yourself if you were truly committed to the change. In most cases, you were not deeply committed. The most powerful reward for change is the elimination of pain. Effective change comes with the realization that you're sick and tired of being sick and tired. Maybe you haven't become disgusted enough yet, or maybe stress and tension haven't affected you enough yet. Or maybe you haven't become agitated enough with resentment and anger to consciously think about changing your self at work.

What is enough? Enough is when you—and only you—decide that conditions—things as they are—aren't working for you. Then you know you're ready to choose something else—something better. Often, it isn't until people become extremely frightened, disgusted, or angry about their own behavior that they can summon enough motivation to carry them through the initial stages of change. Without pain you can experience a heightened awareness of will, mastery, and personal power. That reward becomes very reinforcing.

With those two prerequisites in mind (self-acceptance and a deep desire to change), take some time now to identify what you would like to have more of in your life as a result of reading this book. You may want to flip back through the pages and jot down a checklist of things you want and what you need to change to get them.

Now that you have a list, put a star next to the three items that you are very committed to and then decide which one you will accomplish first. Be sure that what you have chosen is something you want to change. You can use this chapter to help chart your plan to accomplish each area of growth.

"Needing" to change carries with it a heavy burden of obligation; "wanting" to change lightens the load and gives momentum and energy to your motivation for change.

Transition

Linked to change is the process of transition. Transition involves two factors:

1. **Letting go of the old situation and the old identity that went with it.** You can't begin something new until you let go of the old. This phase encompasses "ending." Consider complaining, for example. If you want to stop complaining, you have to let go of more than just the act of complaining. You have to let go of the gratification that comes from complaining, the attention you get, the camaraderie of those who share your complaint, the release of frustration, and so forth. Disengagement from the old has to happen before you can embrace the new.

2. **Passing through the "neutral zone."** Between letting go and making a new beginning, you're in a neutral zone. One example of a neutral zone is adolescence, the period between childhood and adulthood. Another is when new managers, promoted from the ranks of staff nurse, find themselves suddenly confused about their role. You have probably experienced this zone if you've been pulled to another unit. The neutral zone can be a time of confusion, loss, and despair. It is also a time of discovery and reorientation. This takes time. If you recognize that you're in a transition phase—a natural phase—you can live with unsettled feelings knowing that you're on the way to where you want to be.

Attempts to change frequently fail because there is no transition plan. You greatly enhance your ability to make successful changes if you recognize the need for transition and support yourself through the process. This is a time to ask for help from friends and coworkers.

Planned Change versus Unplanned Change

There are two types of change: change that you initiate or control yourself, and change that is "forced" upon you because of a change in your environment. For example:

- **Planned Change: Self-Initiated**
  —Dieting to improve your figure or fit into your clothes
  —Exercising regularly
  —Returning to school or taking a continuing education course
  —Becoming more assertive, especially with a particular doctor

—Finding a new route to work
—Developing new interests
—Managing stress in new ways
- **Unplanned Change: Externally Imposed**
    —Hospital reorganization due to fewer patients, less revenue, or changes in service
    —Death of a friend or relative
    —Computerized order entry systems
    —A promotion
    —Job-related transfers to another state or facility
    —A new nurse manager

Your list of changes probably contains examples of "self-initiated" changes and also changes that have been "externally imposed" upon you. Resistance to change enters into both kinds. But when it comes to externally imposed change, it's especially important to recognize this tendency toward resistance. Thoughts like "they did this to me" or "I didn't ask for it" will block your motivation to make needed change. It may be true that you didn't ask for this or that "they did this to me." However, the decision to embrace the change instead of resisting and resenting it will serve to accelerate, rather than decelerate, the change process. The point is to recognize and to choose. Resistance will only serve to hurt you, not help you.

The Steps in Change

The following 10 steps forward to successful change apply to both planned and unplanned change:

- **Step 1: You become aware of the problem, issue, or situation.** The first step in change is awareness of the need to change. You may recognize this need, or the need for change may be brought to your attention by someone else. At this step, the pressure for change causes tension. Use this tension to help motivate you. Here's an opportunity to use the steps to successful change described in chapter 7, "The How-to's of Working Smarter." Procrastination or avoiding the problem will build tension and create stress. Don't get immobilized.
- **Step 2: Get a clear, concise understanding of what needs to be changed.** Be sure what you define as the problem is the real problem. Is the problem within your control? Is there a possible solution? If you are unsure about your

objectivity, go to step 3. If you are still stuck, ask for help from a friend or colleague.

- **Step 3: Separate your emotional reaction to change from the facts.** Externally imposed changes often generate great emotion, especially anger and defensiveness. Remember that you have choices. Stay out of the Self-Defeating Zone. You are in control of your feelings and reactions. Turn this problem into an opportunity; look for the benefits in the changes you need to make.
- **Step 4: Review your experience with a similar type of problem.** What solutions did you try in the past? Which were successful? Before you eliminate solutions that were unsuccessful, consider their use in this situation.
- **Step 5: Formulate a realistic goal that is stated in behavioral terms and one that you will recognize when you have achieved it.** For example, "I want to lose weight" is much too general. How much weight? How long will it take? How will you know you have achieved it? "I want to lose 10 pounds in two months so that I can fit into these special clothes" is clear and measurable. Your accomplishment is easy to recognize.
- **Step 6: Outline the steps to reach your goal; make a plan.** Remember not to bite off more than you can chew. Make the steps achievable.
- **Step 7: Identify what you might do to undermine your own success in making the needed change.** Know what your own barriers to success are and then commit yourself to removing those barriers. Part of the difficulty in making change is giving up something safe. It doesn't matter if you are dissatisfied with the way things are; change can be more threatening than dissatisfaction with the status quo. So, despite your best efforts, you can undermine your own growth because it is uncomfortable to change. Anyone who has dieted more than once in their lifetime knows this is true.
- **Step 8: Make your move!** Begin the change you have planned.
- **Step 9: Check your progress at regular intervals.** See what's working to achieve your goal. This step also keeps you honest and on target.
- **Step 10: Verify that the change you worked for has been achieved.** Take a good look at what you did to accomplish the change. Enjoy your achievement! Give yourself a reward that supports your change and the efforts you made to reach your goal.

A Trial Run

Your coworker, Sally, comes to work every day and has a list of complaints about the traffic, the weather, her children, staffing, and her assignment. She complains loudly at the nurses' station to incoming staff. The group's morale dips before the night shift ever receives report. You notice that your own optimism is dampened by Sally's behavior.

You recognize that the problem is your *response* to Sally's complaints. You decide to control your own reaction to her. Getting angry at Sally probably won't work to change your morale for the better. In fact, that response didn't help to change either Sally or your attitude last week when you got irritated with her. You also decide not to talk with your coworkers at this point, because you can't control their reactions to Sally.

Your goal is to keep your own outlook positive at the beginning of this day. Instead of listening to Sally, you decide to focus your attention on your patients. In addition to focusing on information you need to plan care for the day, you will silently say to yourself, "There she goes again. Now is the time to refocus and hold onto my positive feelings."

How might you undermine your efforts to achieve your goal? Because you enjoy spending time with other staff, you might hang around the station while Sally complains so that you can be part of the group. But not today. Instead, you decide that for a week you will give up being with the group in the morning and talk with the staff as you work during the day.

You will know you've reached your goal when you still feel positive as you finish report. At the end of the week, you find that you have been able to stay positive and haven't allowed yourself to be drawn into complaints. You are encouraged and decide to talk with Sally about her behavior. A guide to change is presented in figure 9-1. Try using it the next time you plan a change.

Figure 9-1. Guide to Change

1. What is the problem, issue, or situation?
2. What needs to change? Do you control that? If not, who does?
3. When you think about needing to make this change, what do you feel? What do you need to let go of? What are you losing or gaining?
4. Plan what you need to do to support yourself.
5. Have you confronted this *problem* (or its solution) before? What did you do? What was the result?
6. What is your goal? Keep it simple and behavioral.
7. What do you need to do to reach your goal?
8. What might you do to sabotage your efforts to change? How can you catch yourself?
9. How will you evaluate your progress?

Change: The Process

Before you begin working on your first area of growth, remember how long it has taken you to become good at the old thought or action. Change doesn't happen overnight, either. Here is a very common course the change process takes:

1. **"Oops, I did it again."** The first step in change is the hindsight that you responded with the old behavior again. The recognition process is very important; it occurs after the fact in the beginning of change. Give yourself a pat on the back.
2. **"Look, I'm doing it now."** The next step in change is seeing yourself responding with the old behavior while you are doing it. You even continue to do it. Don't get upset. You have made progress! Now you are recognizing your old behavior while you're doing it, not after the fact. Pat yourself on the back.
3. **"Look, I'm doing it now, and I want to back up and start over."** The growth is obvious. Give yourself a big hug!
4. **"Here comes a situation where I would respond with the old behavior."** In most cases, you will use the new behavior. Tell yourself how wonderful you are.
5. **"Say, I just responded with the new behavior without thinking about it!"** What reward could you give yourself for accomplishing this much growth? Give it to yourself!
6. **"Oops, I used the old behavior again."** Even after you use the new behavior automatically, you will occasionally slip back and use the old behavior. Growth and change are a lifelong process that seldom ends with perfection. Give yourself a cheer for your success and effort!

Additional Tips for Success

Here are tips that can help you anticipate positive results when you make changes:

- **Pat yourself on the back for your effort.** Even if you don't accomplish what you want on the first or second try, you made the effort to face the issue and take responsibility for your life. Think of the number of experiments Thomas Edison conducted before he invented the light bulb. It was over 200!
- **If you feel stuck, try to reframe the situation or change your perception of the problem.** See the glass as half full,

not half empty. Remember when we mentioned the example of the wealthy patient who had been described in the change-of-shift report as demanding and irritable? We decided that she was probably threatened by her illness; her irritability was her attempt to cope.

- **Check out your assumptions about the problem or facts.** It is often your assumptions about the problem that prevent you from finding a solution. For example, let's say several procedures on your unit are changed. Some of the staff seem to know about the changes, but no one informed you. You could assume that people don't like you, or that your nurse manager doesn't value you and neglects to tell you about things. These assumptions prevent you from finding out the information you need to give care appropriately and could stop you from getting information in the future. In fact, the changes were announced at a staff meeting while you were on vacation. You are unaware that minutes from all staff meetings are posted on the bulletin board.
- **Make small changes in what you do by trying out new behaviors.** This will help to lessen your dread of change. You could sit in a new chair in staff meetings, try a different route home, or try a new response when the linen is late.
- **Remember to attempt to change only what you have some control over.** Nurses report feeling responsible for *everything* that happens to patients while having little control over many of the factors that meet patient needs (for example, linen, food, medications, exam trays, visitors, and information). Bedside nurses need to work with their head nurse or nurse managers to change problems that involve other departments.
- **Pick your priorities.** It's hard to change many things at once. A concentrated effort in one direction is likely to effect greater results. You may gain greater perspective on your priorities if you select your high-priority changes in light of your professional/personal goals. Which changes move you forward in your process of personal/professional growth?
- **Ask for help when you get stuck.**

Summary

This chapter has described change as an opportunity for growth and how to escape the web of resistance we are all so good at constructing. We have discussed the process of change and why it is so necessary to have a transition plan to create the changes you most desire. We all want to act on the things we know are good for us. We hope that you have many more skills and ideas about how to successfully support yourself in the change process so you can make it as joyful and exciting as possible. Become a lover of changes and a pursuer of growth; it will keep you healthy and happy.

Epilogue

We hope this book has made you aware of the many choices you have in your daily life as a nurse. The kinds of choices we've been talking about are not the ones you would make with the toss of a coin, but rather the basic, long-term choices you as a nurse must recommit to every single day. These are life choices that open you to all the potential power and happiness of your life and your chosen career. We hope this book has given you not only the insights and tools to rescue yourself from those "bad days," but also the means to soar like an eagle—to be everything you want yourself to be. It's exhilarating—and a bit scary—to know once and for all that your job satisfaction and well-being are your responsibility.

As you know, there is no greater source of meaning and gratification in life than helping others and caring for others. But in order to care for others, you must first take care of yourself. And that's one lesson in life in which you need to be able to step back and honestly say, "I've learned that one!"

We hope we've helped you to do this. And here's our final wish for you:

> Be your own very best friend, make an *all-out commitment* to your own happiness, and realize every day the richness of your experience as a nurse and the beauty of your profession.

Thank you for making this journey with us. And most of all, on behalf of *all* patients, thank you for choosing to be a nurse—a nurse dedicated to professional growth and personal happiness. We salute you, and we wish you harmony in your life, always.

Appendix

Harmony Self-Appraisal

R ead each of the statements listed below and consider how each applies to you. Then circle one of the numbers at the far right of that statement, ranging from "Almost All of the Time" to "Almost Never." Take your time with each statement and feel how strongly it applies to you.

	Almost All of the Time	Much of the Time	Sometimes	Not Often	Almost Never
1. **Positive Mind-Set**					
a. I am full of hope and optimism, not weighed down with fear and pessimism	5	4	3	2	1
b. I am at ease; I keep frustration and annoyance to a minimum.	5	4	3	2	1
c. I value high achievement standards; I do not allow them to be a source of stress.	5	4	3	2	1
d. I am content with where I am in life. If I become restless, I know I have choices that I can act on.	5	4	3	2	1

	Almost All of the Time	Much of the Time	Sometimes	Not Often	Almost Never
e. I go with the flow of the river of life and let go easily of what I cannot control.	5	4	3	2	1
2. Positive Feelings					
a. I feel very secure; I experience little jealousy or competition.	5	4	3	2	1
b. I feel confident and empowered to accomplish what I choose in life.	5	4	3	2	1
c. I am peaceful and free of guilt and worry.	5	4	3	2	1
d. I consciously choose my feelings.	5	4	3	2	1
e. I am able to quickly let go of negative feelings of my own and of others.	5	4	3	2	1
3. Positive Energy					
a. I have a high level of physical energy through-out the workday.	5	4	3	2	1
b. I am emotionally available for my patients when I am with them.	5	4	3	2	1
c. I find myself challenged and stimulated by my work. I don't feel stagnated or bored.	5	4	3	2	1

	Almost All of the Time	Much of the Time	Sometimes	Not Often	Almost Never
d. Taking initiative to solve problems is something I do readily and easily.	5	4	3	2	1
e. I find an abundance of reward and recognition in my work.	5	4	3	2	1
4. Personal Power					
a. I am mobilized to work for improvement and change within the system; I don't feel defeated or helpless.	5	4	3	2	1
b. I take responsibility for my own job satisfaction and success. I don't blame others.	5	4	3	2	1
c. I feel empowered to influence decisions and affect change.	5	4	3	2	1
d. My self-esteem is high.	5	4	3	2	1
e. I am genuinely focused on and concerned about others when I am with them; I don't feel the need to voice my own achievements.	5	4	3	2	1

	Almost All of the Time	Much of the Time	Sometimes	Not Often	Almost Never
5. Positive Work Relationships					
a. I feel open and accepting toward my coworkers and feel free of hidden resentments and bitterness.	5	4	3	2	1
b. I view conflict as inevitable and healthy, and I approach it in an open, problem-solving manner with others.	5	4	3	2	1
c. I feel a strong sense of belonging in my workplace.	5	4	3	2	1
d. I communicate openly and effectively with others.	5	4	3	2	1
e. I make it comfortable for others to give me feedback. I am receptive and responsive.	5	4	3	2	1
6. Positive Patient Care					
a. I am able to get a lot done without giving the impression that I'm too busy to listen and respond to patient needs.	5	4	3	2	1

	Almost All of the Time	Much of the Time	Sometimes	Not Often	Almost Never
b. I make it a high priority to establish positive rapport with my patients; I see the person behind the patient.	5	4	3	2	1
c. I'm pleasant at the bedside without appearing to be hassled, irritated, or moody.	5	4	3	2	1
d. I keep my clinical skills at peak.	5	4	3	2	1
e. Behind the scenes I treat patient care issues with respect and dignity; I don't give in to negative, cynical, and dehumanizing attitudes.	5	4	3	2	1

7. **Skills and Abilities**

a. I can handle multiple demands skillfully. I don't get anxious or overwhelmed.	5	4	3	2	1
b. I am realistic about what I can do, and I don't get caught up in the frustration of unrealistic self-expectations.	5	4	3	2	1

	Almost All of the Time	Much of the Time	Sometimes	Not Often	Almost Never
c. I am able to say no without feeling obligated and guilty.	5	4	3	2	1
d. I am resourceful and creative in solving problems.	5	4	3	2	1
e. I am able to assert myself effectively and have little problem with being passive or aggressive in my style.	5	4	3	2	1

8. **Personal-Professional Balance**

	Almost All of the Time	Much of the Time	Sometimes	Not Often	Almost Never
a. I can disengage and leave work at work and fully participate in my outside life.	5	4	3	2	1
b. My home life is happy and harmonious.	5	4	3	2	1
c. I have energy to use my free time creatively.	5	4	3	2	1
d. I feel a balance between my professional role and my personal life and responsibilities.	5	4	3	2	1
e. I am successful in finding quality time just for me when I can renew my own sense of self.	5	4	3	2	1

	Almost All of the Time	Much of the Time	Sometimes	Not Often	Almost Never
9. Health and Well-Being					
a. I feel fit, energetic, and healthy.	5	4	3	2	1
b. I have no physical signs or symptoms of illness.	5	4	3	2	1
c. I sleep well; I need no help in falling asleep.	5	4	3	2	1
d. I engage in vigorous physical exercise at least three times a week.	5	4	3	2	1
e. I eat with health in mind. I choose wholesome foods.	5	4	3	2	1

Overall Reaction to the Harmony Self-Appraisal

Of the four statements listed below, select the one that best describes your dominant thoughts while filling out the Harmony Self-Appraisal. If no alternative describes your thoughts exactly, just zero in on the closest one.

☐ I'll bet my score will be high because I work hard at being healthy in mind and body. Also, I pride myself on being good at what I do as a nurse.

☐ I'll probably score high on some questions and not so high on others. That's OK because my main concern is learning more about myself.

☐ I hope my score is decent. It makes me anxious when I think I'm not doing well.

☐ I hate these things. I'll probably score so low that I'll embarrass myself. Then I'll end up feeling awful. Maybe I shouldn't bother filling it out.

How to Interpret Your Score

Only you can interpret your score. There is no score that is good or bad, high or low. The purpose of this self-test is threefold—it is meant to help you accomplish the following:

- Look at yourself more closely.
- Gain personal clarity about where you are.
- Identify factors working for you and against you in your quest for fulfillment and well-being in your life and work.

So why use the numbering system? It's there to provide a baseline score for yourself. Then you can check on your own progress as you integrate the principles and skills described in this book. Compare your score now with your score later. Take a new look every three to six months to see how far you've progressed:

- Am I satisfied with my overall results?
- How satisfied am I with my answers in each section?
- Which areas stand out as meriting special attention or adjustment?
- What are my priority areas for further work?
- What's blocking me from making the changes I want?
- What am I willing to do to make desired changes?

Your outlook is more important than your score. Unfortunately, people tend to dwell on their inadequacies more than their strengths. In the spirit of Harmony, it would be helpful to avoid doing this. Think to yourself:

In some areas, I'm doing okay. In some, I'm doing great. In others, I haven't yet begun to develop myself. Yesterday is history. What matters is what I do with today and tomorrow. Just because I was a certain way yesterday does not mean I can't be different today. Stretching and growing is what life's about. I welcome the chance to learn more about myself. Who said I had to be the perfect nurse, anyway?

Right now, go back and read the above self-talk five times. *Imprint* these healthy thoughts into your brain. You can *choose* to think what you want to think. You're in control, so take charge!